TABLE TONICS

A Beginner's Guide

To Botanical Medicine

For Strength, Balance

and Longevity

Peter Sundance

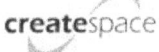

createspace

Library Reference Data
Sundance, Peter.
Table tonics. / Peter Sundance. 1st ed.
Includes references.
1. Health. 2. Physical fitness. 3. Longevity. I. Title.
II. Title: Table Tonics
ISBN-13: 978-1-535-03618-4

All illustrations by Peter Sundance.

Thank you farmers, drivers and merchants who make today's food system run around the clock. Thank you teachers, professionals, parents, and students who actively look for new ways to solve old problems. Thank you Mom and Dad for living your lives and letting me play drums on everything.
Thank you Earth.

tonic: (1) a medicinal substance that brings health and prosperity, (2) the leading tone (backbone) in a musical arrangement.

We need the tonic of wilderness. We are earnest to explore and learn all things, and we require that all things be **mysterious** and **unexplorable**, that land and sea be **infinitely wild.** We are witnessing our own limits transgressed, and remember the life pasturing freely where we never wander.

From *Walden* by Henry David Thoreau

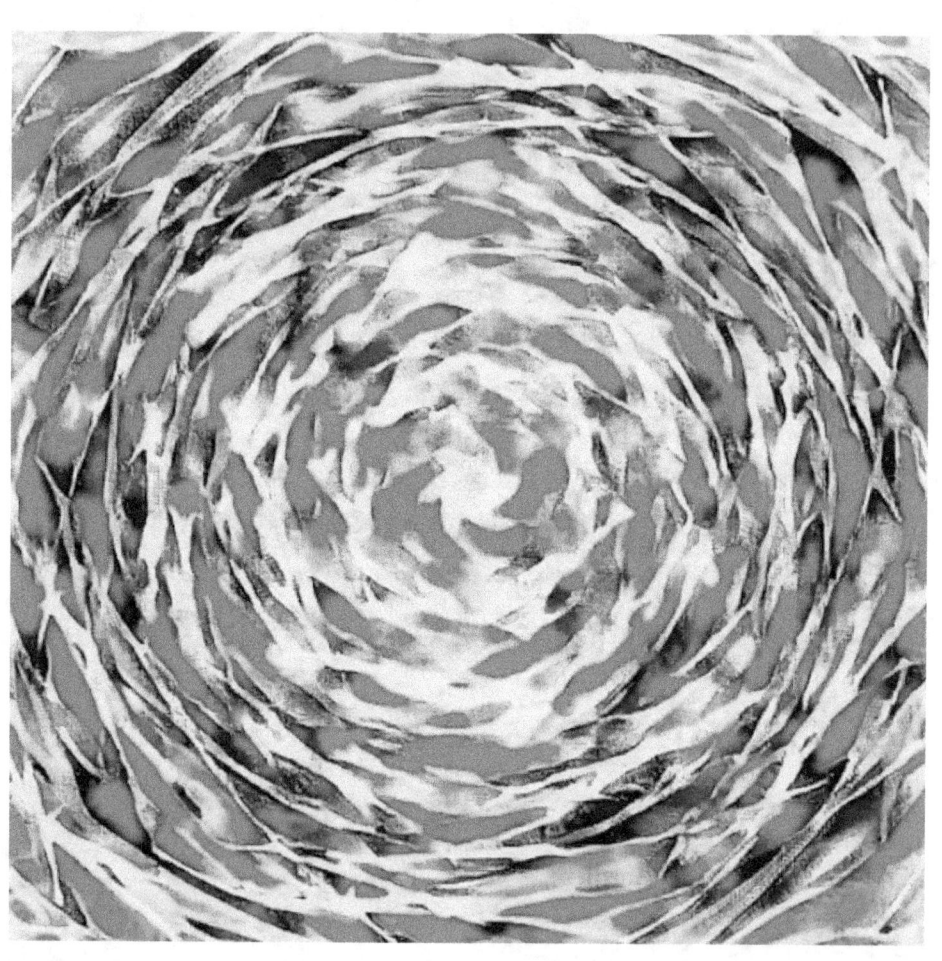

Table of Contents

Three: Natural Science

Welcome

This step-by-step "How To" Guide shares instructions for life success in fitness, productivity and vibrant health - through the raw, unfiltered energy of Mother Earth.

This is an Introduction to Natural Living Arts, an expressive method of Stress Management. You will craft fine experiences with the organic meals and home-brewed Elixirs in this book – and learn to innovate in the process.

Learn to apply ageless practices that harness biological phenomena – enhancing our ability to engage in life's myriad of daily adventures.

We connect to the source of vitality, the seed of life, at home and wherever we go, with direct guidance to explore this land where we work, play and dream together.

Be happy you are here!

About this Book

This is a manual for how to manage energy – by coming together around real food. This handbook sources fresh, nutrient-dense, quality ingredients (*functional foods*) allowing you to feel light and full of energy.

Functional foods give us "tone" to our bodies (you can think of it as a musical note) which supports physical mobility and mental alertness. You are the instrument, letting the Earth play her harmonies through you.

You and your loved ones may notice a vibrant energy from making the elixirs and meals in this manual on a daily basis. Functional foods represent the love of the Earth for us, bringing great wealth beyond words.

Fresh = Functional

The recipes in this book (planets) orbit around the idea that <u>fresh food is functional food</u> (the sun).

Many foods are excluded from this manual, specifically any pre-made food, to show the simplicity of making meals with single-ingredient foods from scratch. This way of living requires a search for variety within specific limitations. We use home recipes to help the average person transition to meals rich in whole foods. This manual includes some animal products and it excludes animal flesh on the ethical principle of "live and let live." We obtain the essential nutrients from functional foods.

In general, your best bet for optimum nourishment involves living an active life, primarily so that you are hungry and eat functional foods that provide the essential nutrients. You may notice less hunger which can mean your body is "full" of nutrients, and requires smaller amounts of these same foods. For specific questions, you can ask your Primary Care Physician (MD) to discuss nutrition with you and refer you to a qualified healthcare practitioner: a Nutritionist (RD), Personal Trainer (CPT), Naturopathic Doctor (ND).

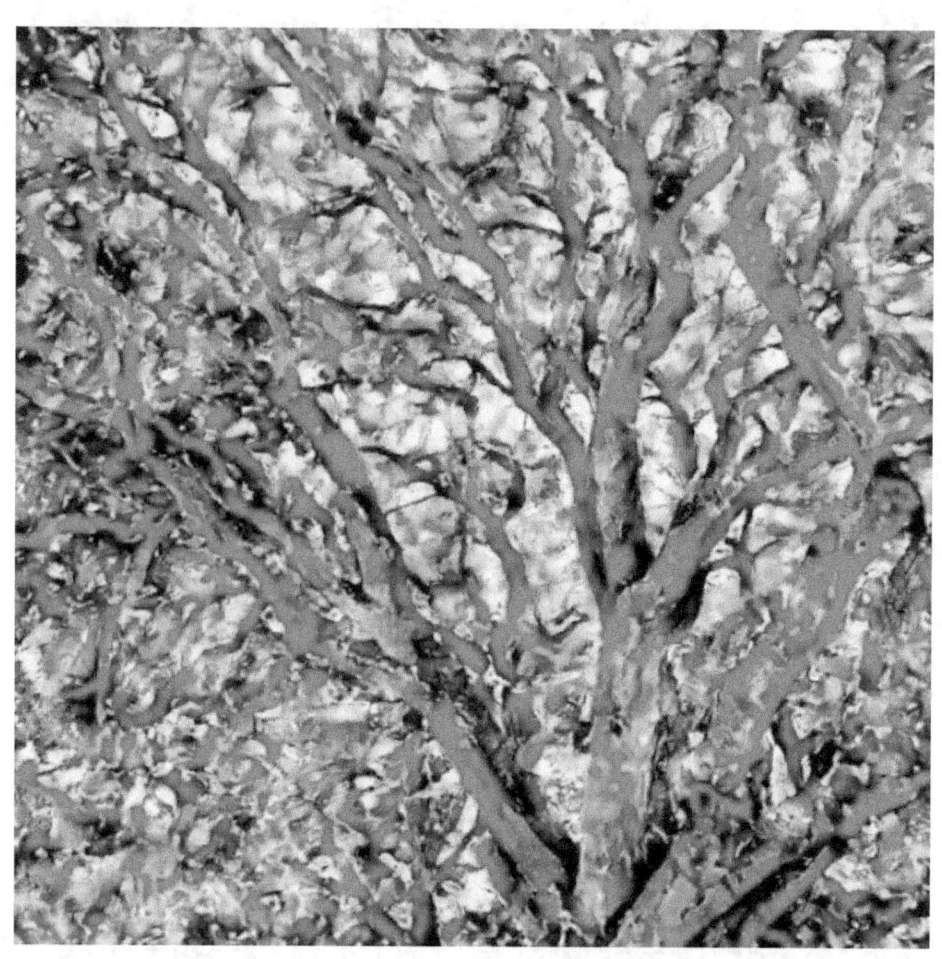

We start by exploring the connections between ourselves and our world. This gives us food for thought, chew on these ideas, and savor the flavor.

The body is the kingdom. You are the ruler. You bring happiness and prosperity to your land. You lead by example, which gains the respect of other rulers. This respect brings cooperation. Everyone has a cooperation celebration. Life is awesome.

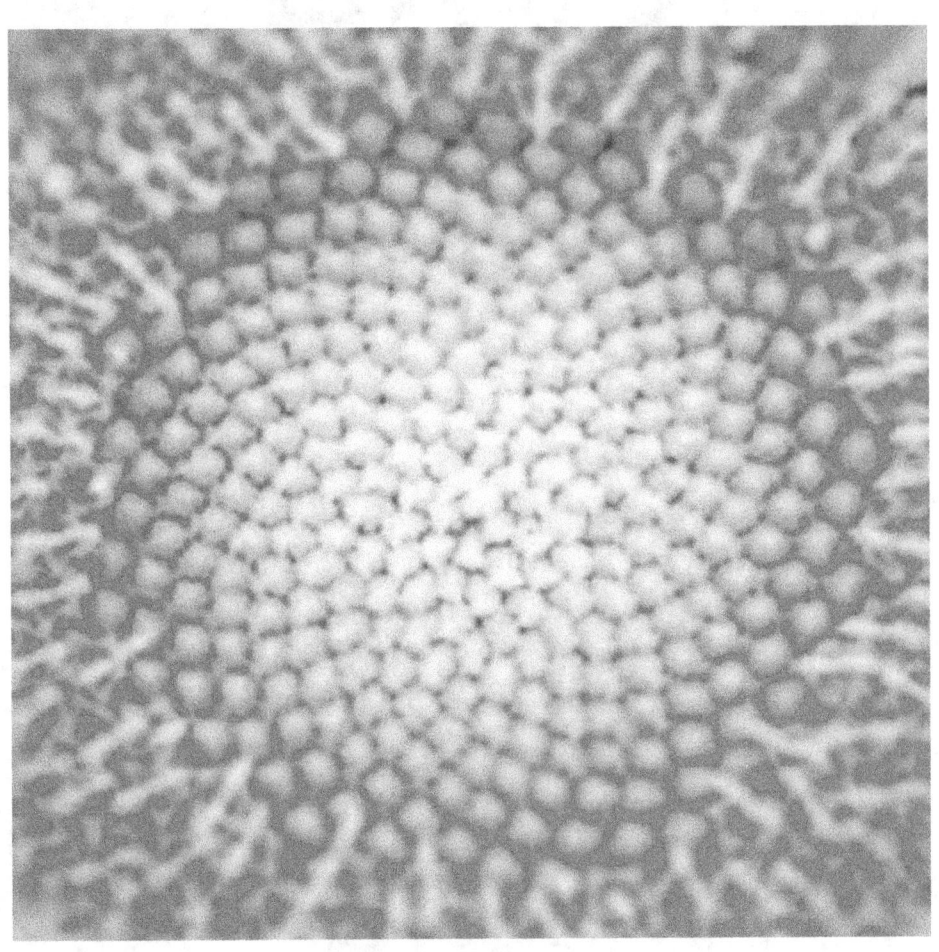

One

Vital Functions

Simplicity

Save time, be happy.

This manual provides One-Step Recipes to rejuvenate you and your family with unique combinations of common single-ingredient foods available at many grocery stores. Every ingredient has a function - to provide you with a burning energy to live life.

In places with limited fresh produce, garden and sprout foods to save money and increase your bounty. For bulk non-perishables, such as spices, herbs, grains, seeds, nuts and legumes - you can find organic versions of these online at wholesale prices.

The One-Step Recipes save time, energy, and space in your memory. You will have less dishes to wash and more time to enjoy the people you love. Many instances call for chopped foods, which you can prepare in large batches on a weekly basis (on laundry day). See the Resources Guide for further reading.

Again, this manual simplifies many practices into one main idea: fresh food is functional. Fun is functional too. So have some, on this adventure into the great unknown.

Access

This is a hallmark of a successful community, and a proverbial "elephant in the room" when it comes to the discussion of equality and human rights. Public access to fresh quality ingredients ensures the health of people and the land. In the cycle of life, quality food requires quality soil, which requires that we who take from the land treat it with respect in order to continue our use of it. This interaction ensures that soil (as well as water and air) remains healthy and arable for generations. In order to maintain healthy land, we support systems that sustain us. Biodynamic (organic) farming forms a foundations for food access by recycling nutrients (through composting and seasonal crop rotation), saving seeds from year to year, and connecting us with the land on a daily basis to guarantee quality.

Currently, the world produces enough food to sustain a population of 10 billion people. Even in "modern" nations, we see problems of food access due to income, education, and time. A simple fix (that takes time and energy): Grow your own (potted tomatoes on a window sill, sprouts in a jar, curbside community garden patch). The world is naturally abundant, even in urban "food deserts" you can find patches of wild dandelion greens growing out of sidewalks. It is clear that the mass distribution of food products can trifle with our notion of convenience, because the quality we sacrifice for time is worth more than gold. Quality food prepared with care can relieve symptoms of major illnesses and provide means for an active, peaceful life. We can have convenience and quality, and replace a hunger for instant gratification with a satisfaction that's rooted in understanding the earth.

Success

Sharing fresh food with your family

Expressing your inner muse by crafting a fine-dining experience

Supporting a socially just world

Making meals with minimal effort, maximum nutrition and flavor

Connecting to the physical world in a living exchange of energy

Saving time and money

Success: Your First Recipe

Serves Everyone

Prep Time: 5 minutes

Ingredients:

This Handbook

Intuition

Determination

A Goal

A Friend

Instructions:

Combine the essential ingredients for success. Achieve success.

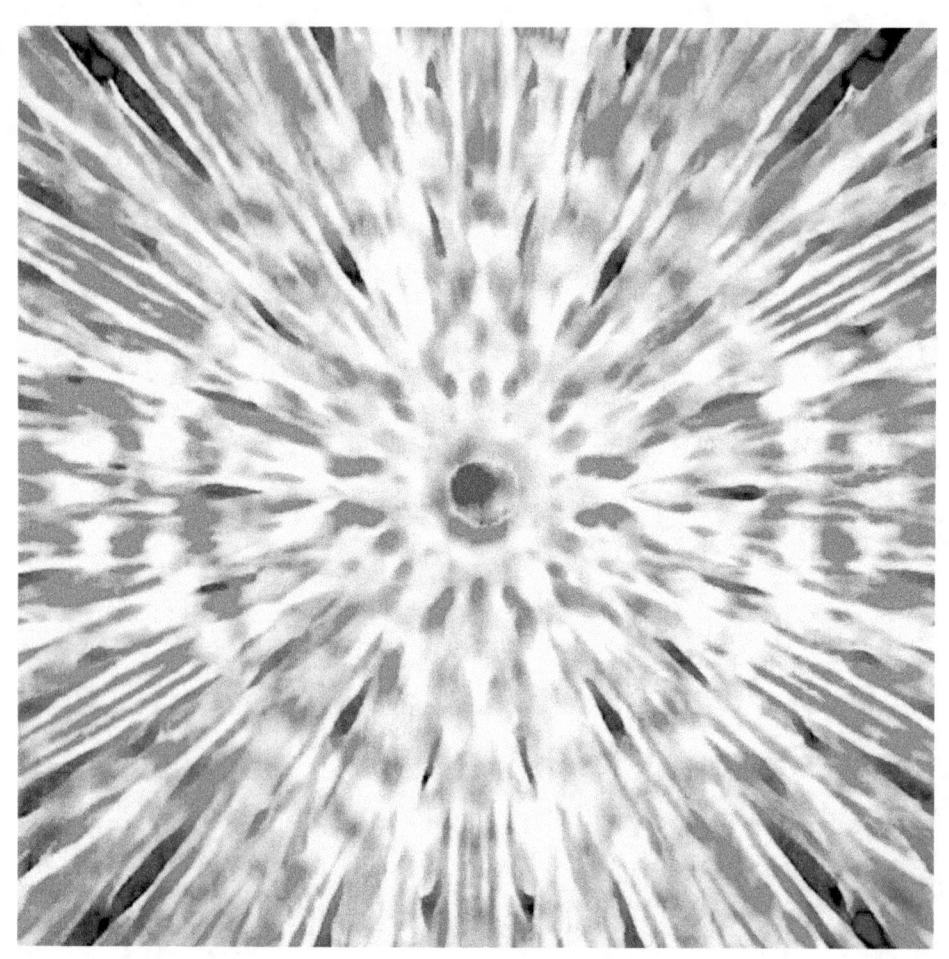

The Idea: Fresh=Functional

Why: In every corner of the world, humankind strives to perfect the craft of making food. Functional food provides a bounty of nourishment to sustain our lives. Eating is as necessary of a human activity as sleeping and laughing. We come together around the meals we share. By coming together, we support the land, farmers, and communities, creating mutual benefits through the entire cycle of life.

How: This Manual provides you with ancient principles, practical science, kitchen basics, recipes, grocery checklists, quick tips and resources to get you started.

What: You are a master builder, you can make what you imagine.

Five Functions of Fresh

1: Investing in Yourself

Supporting yourself with fresh foods supports farmers who take care of the land, and ensure that quality food stays on the table. Small-scale farmers make up 80% of all the organic food grown in this country and you can ask these people who produce the food exactly how it grows. Go to *localharvest.org* for a list of farm delivery services (CSAs) and farmers markets.

2: Mixing it Up

Varying the type of fresh foods you eat allows your body to maintain a vibrant, dynamic community of bacteria in your stomach designed to break down many different kinds of foods. In the stomach alone, 100 trillion "healthy" bacteria, about 3 pounds worth, digest food for us and help us respond effectively to illness. These bacteria (pre- and pro-biotics) come from the ground and are essential for us to live, be active and think clearly. *Eating foods in-season helps us maintain this variety.*

3: Vitamin Earth

We connect the health of the earth and the health of ourselves together to see a clear picture of how to live functionally. Those 100 trillion bacteria in our stomach come from healthy dirt that grows fresh food. We require quality water, air, and soil to bring us the vital energy that lets us live here.

4: Using Your Gut Instinct

This statement can apply to most of life. Foods processed with chemicals, as well as many medications such as antibiotics and steroids, can change the balance of the probiotic bacteria that protect us from illness. In fact, 90% of all the serotonin (a molecule responsible for happiness and sleep) is produced in the gut.

5: Getting to Garden

Time on a farm and in a garden can give you a new perspective on the life cycles that we take part in. It can help us learn how to look at life up-close and as a whole system, and gives us a chance to socialize and ask questions about how systems work. We learn how to gain freedom in an interdependent system.

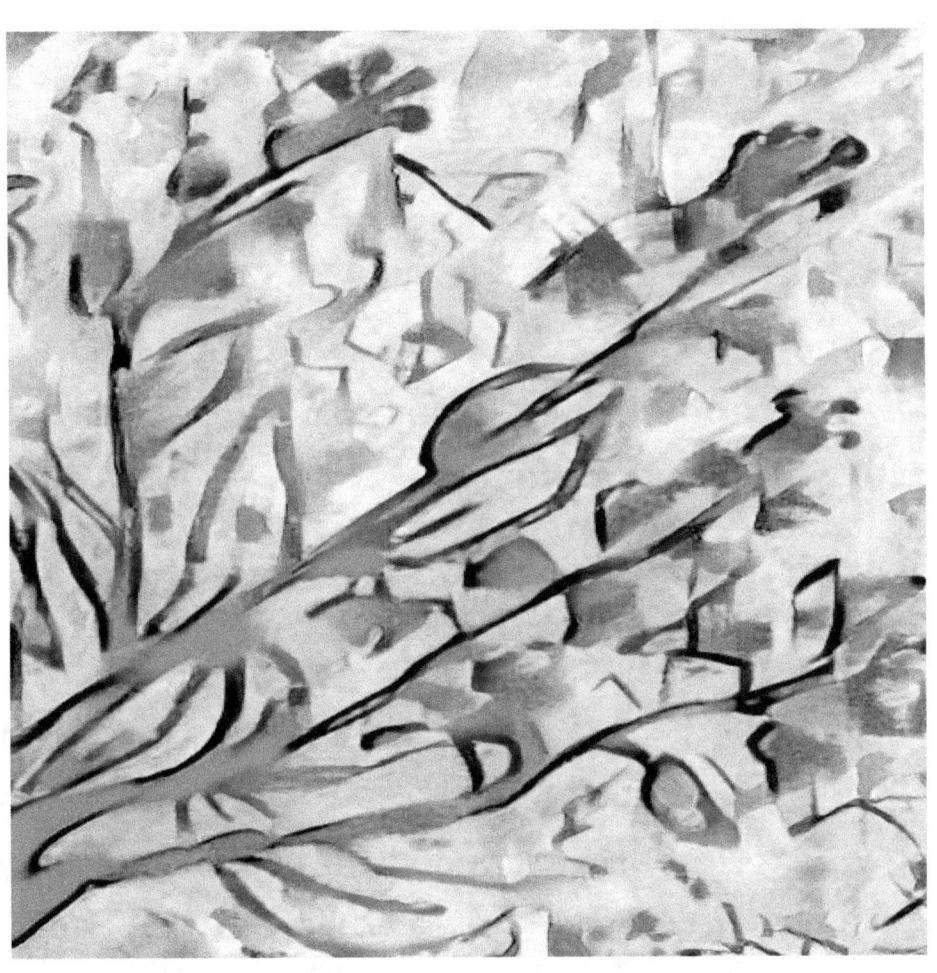

We are Dirt

dirt is earth. it is alive in you and I.

is it nature to be this way?

how do we stay close? how do we play?

how do we make sense of the earth?

always rebalancing, where do we sink our roots and soak up the sun?

how do we make our short lives last?

and enjoy every morning dew drop?

why do we need what we need?

how do we talk to each other? how many seasons will we see? how do we open up and flower and let life perpetuate life?

in the mystic cycle, we smell the dirt, we are dirt.

A Universal Perspective

Everything comes from a single source. Call it what you want. A point. Now, that single point is the entire universe. And it's getting bigger all the time, it's still one universe that started from one point. Personal awareness works the same way. You are the ever-expanding universe. Everyday you can learn something new, and your personal universe grows. So, how do you learn how to learn?

We can maintain an open outlook to the world by observing new ideas from a distance. Ultimately, we are susceptible to the universal patterns that form our genetic instincts and learning behavior. We can learn from these patterns to make decisions.

Historically, "rational thinking" is a new concept. In our primal ancestors of ten million years ago, imagine the first communication of ideas including hungry, horny, scary, and sleepy for the purpose of species survival. Scientific records indicate that our ancestral diet consisted of mostly leaves, with some fruit, fungus, bugs and a bird now and again.

Conveniently, in today's world, people can decide what to eat and when to eat it. This luxury allows people to experience a full spectrum of foods. In turn, we give our life to a food through eating, and the opposite holds true as well.

Our understanding of evolution shows how we can live on almost anything. I believe every *individual* has an optimal diet, and it can change over time. For all people, a simple variety of mostly plant-based, farm fresh, tasty food gets the job done well.

Believe in your experience, and follow it to where you need to go. Remember, you are a living, breathing child of the universe (the atoms that make up all of Planet Earth were fused at the center of a star going supernova).

You have a reason for reading this. You can educate yourself and know yourself to see beyond culturally imposed ideas from people and books. You can use the limits of your body as a guide for sensing a way of living that is in harmony with nature. This book guides you through this experience with One-Step Recipes made from fresh food.

Materializing Mood

Food = Energy = Emotions = Body = World

We enhance the body's natural ability to turn food into enjoyment by choosing to eat fresh food in a fresh mood. You define that mood for yourself. Every day is a fresh start, a chance to think, feel, and act in way that brings us into a place of space, where we can explore and remember and change freely.

We limit ourselves through our ability to decide what we can do. We can make one simple decision - to enjoy whatever we are doing at this transitory crossroads in space-time. You can now decide what you want to learn from the world, how you will spend your time, and bring a fresh perspective wherever you go.

3 Steps to a Fresh Mood

1. Say to yourself, *"I am in harmony with nature"* to stay on track.

2. Take 5 minutes to picture your ideal life, breathing out with the old and in with the new.

3. Remind yourself to work towards this goal daily.

Accepting Attention

Staying calm is a method for keeping the mind alert and open to all that's around. Engaging this idea, you can come close to yourself by letting life work in your favor. You can observe the rules you impose upon yourself and make note of how you are living moment to moment. This is smelling fresh-cut herbs, this is reflecting, this is watching steam pour from a pot of tea, this is tracking fitness, this is journaling, this is sitting down with a close friend and discussing what's going on in life.

You can begin to notice how the imagination works, and makes a story for life, including the immediate present of "this is happening and this is how I am responding" and the personal narrative of "this is where I've been, this is where I'm going." You can see how life is up to you, and the choices you make are intimately connected to everything around you. So much of life is out of your control, your actions are up to you. Fresh food is calm. Calm is peace. That's why staying calm is key. It's one way that you can bring peace to the world in everyday life.

Electrifying Earth

Being grounded means connecting to our bodies as they relate to the world of people and places and actions. We can often times be pulled from experiencing our bodies. We experience ideas (this paragraph for example) which can bring us out of our bodies and into a state of existence free from the physical world, to some degree.

We can come back to sensing our bodies in many ways. Right now, you can do this by paying attention to your posture, heartbeat and breathing.

Interpreting and applying ideas is a learning process that produces a physical effect. As living organisms, our bodies constantly give and receive feedback from the environment, mainly to keep us in a state of biological homeostasis that we know by different names: happy, alive, balanced, peaceful, satisfied.

The idea of grounding tunes us into the electrical nature of ourselves. For example, the human brain fires electrical impulses at an astronomical rate (more than a trillion times per second). Our highly-charged nature makes it vital for us to connect that electricity to the Earth, which helps us maintain that ebb and flow of energy in the physical world, like plants rooting into the soil for strength. You can always dig your hands straight into the dirt and see what kind of *subterrestrial life forms* are living under your feet (avoid eating worms, as they promote soil diversity).

Ways to Earth

Paying attention to your posture, heartbeat and breathing.

Going for a nature walk.

Limiting time indoors and on electronics.

Connecting to your food source – gardening, farming, preparing real food.

Sharing experiences – especially meals and activities – with the people you love.

Playing games, doing martial arts and activities outdoors.

Camping.

Your Earthy activities:

_____

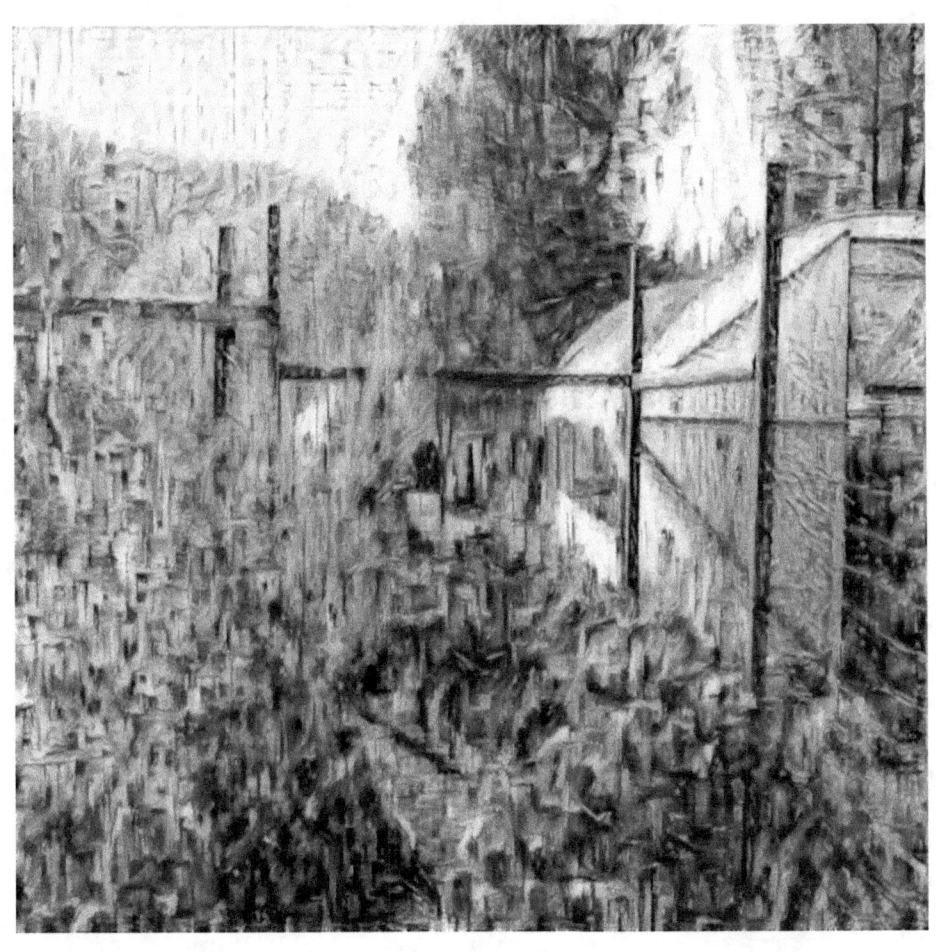

Functional Food Principles

Affordable:

Time and Cost Efficient

Readily Available

Simple and Social

Tasty:

Satisfying to All Five Senses

Varied Texture and Flavor

Vital:

Mostly Plants

Low Glycemic Carbohydrates, Unrefined Fats, Lean Proteins

Free of cow dairy products, additives, processing agents, refined ("white") sugars/grains and preservatives

Balanced ratio of Macronutrients and
   Micronutrients

Humane:

Certified "Fair-Trade" and "Organic"
   (Pesticide Free)

Wild/Grass-fed/Cage-
   free/Kosher/Halal/Local Animal Products

Local Produce (Small Scale Farms/Farmer's
   Markets)

A Humane Food System

"Nothing will benefit human health and increase the chances for survival of life on earth as much as the evolution to a vegetarian diet." - Albert Einstein

Keyword: evolution. This is an ongoing process and every action counts. The greater change that we make, the greater change we will see. Also, plants make energy from sunlight, so the more plants you eat, the more sunlight you eat, and sunlight is very filling.

The term "humane" denotes respect. This includes respect for the land, the workers, and animals. Specifically, this means (a) appreciating and using all of what we take from the land, (b) providing clean, spacious environments for farm animals to live quality lives, and (c) guaranteeing transparency in the food production cycle including growing, processing, and labeling.

We support fresh, functional food in order to support ourselves and the land we live on. This is a way of life, thank you for doing what you can.

Food and Identity

We are creatures with an evolutionary history of omnivory - limited to what's on the ground, in the water, and flying in the air. This Earth is our homeland. It gives us simple choices for what to have for breakfast. In our current society, we can let our social group influence these choices, which helps us contextualize an identity for ourselves.

An identity helps us live in a coherent way. Making a salad from the organic farmland you tend to, ordering a sandwich, catching a fish, and going out for Thai food all require an interaction, in a specific setting, to obtain those meals, which produces a given experience. Through socializing, we incorporate ourselves into systems that support us, feed us, and create a sense of connectedness. Our food is a catalyst that allows us to paint our identity into the frame of the world - a painting of our personal story, a physical body and a community.

We incorporate foods into our bodies, people into our lives, and experiences into our memories. At best, we savor the flavor, even your friend's "experimental" broccoli-peanut butter smoothie.

Fresh Food Defined

Fresh = Bright Colors = Nutritious = Flavor = Quality

Close to the Source

Ultimate Freshness = Harvesting, preparing and eating food in the same day.

Prepared food stays fresh for 24 hours when refrigerated.

Fresh food comes from fresh dirt. You can find fresh dirt everywhere that trees grow and birds sing.

Local farmers and the internet can help you get started with a home garden.

In general, quality food comes from a verifiable source, such as a farmer you can talk to.

Verification: Certified Organic

USDA, EU, and QAI place a seal of approval on "organically" farmed foods.

Visit this site for US Standards:
http://bit.ly/2aeP4cB

In general, the term "organic" farming means that farmers (a) support animal welfare, (b) conserve resources and (c) use natural (non-synthetic/non-GMO) fertilizers, pesticides and seeds to maintain biological balance.

Organic does not guarantee that food is local, humane, and good for you. Food products must be 95% organic to be labeled "Certified Organic." A topic of debate, studies show that organic and conventionally grown produce have comparable nutrient values. Local, organic food has better flavor. The gophers, deer and rabbits can tell you all about it.

Global Subsistence Practices

1. *Farming-Hunting-Foraging*
Growing, catching and finding food
2. *Ordering Out*
Paying someone to make food for you
because it saves time and energy
3. *Dieting*
Prescribing oneself to a specific food pattern
for a range of purposes
4. *Fasting*
Restricting caloric intake for a period of time
5. *Feasting*
Indulging the senses
6. *Cooking for Yourself*
Preparing meals from scratch
7. *Doing What It Takes*
Keeping yourself alive

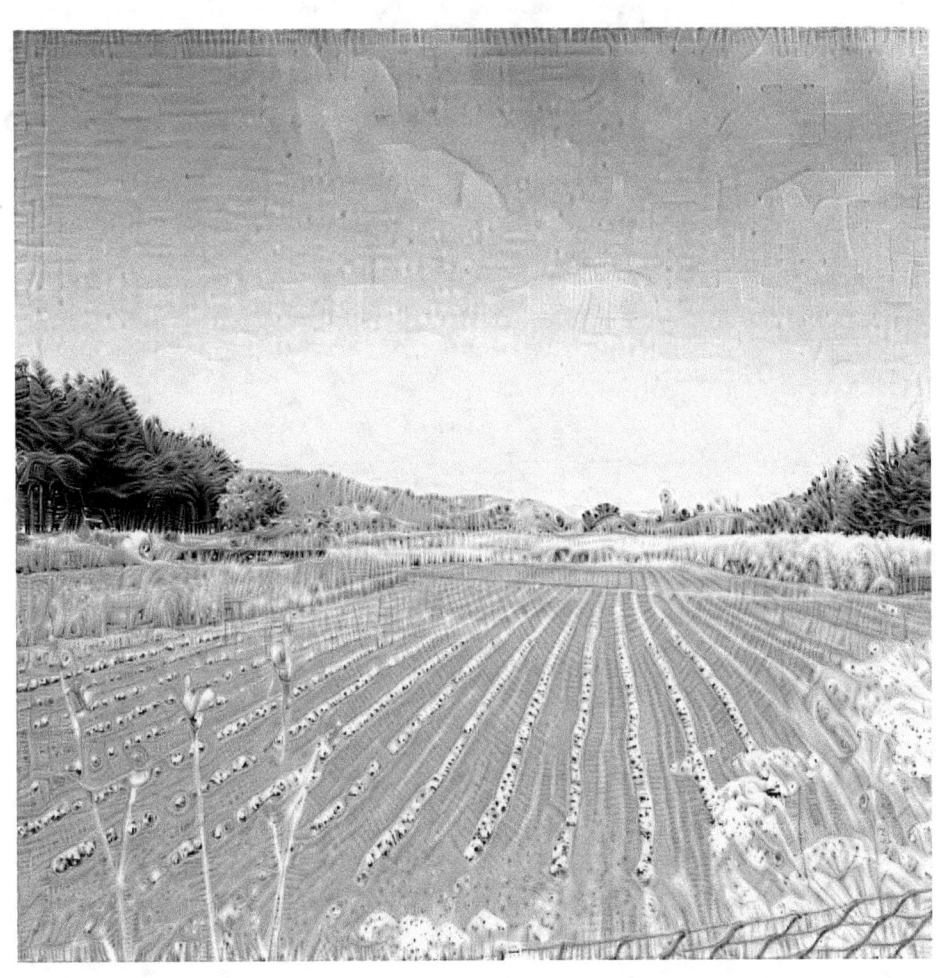

Two

How-To

How to Give That Fresh Feeling

You can find fresh food in many places, from the local produce stand to the herbs growing on the side of the road. These are ways to simplify the process of bringing fresh food into your life.

Working a home garden/organic farm: wwoof.org

Tracking what you eat in a food journal

Making food at home (steam, sun-fry, sprout)

Buying organic food in bulk with friends to save money

Finding food in a local park/forest, especially dandelions

Going to Farmer's Markets/farm stands: localharvest.org

Signing up for a local CSA Program: localharvest.org (again)

Supporting food co-operatives strongertogether.coop

Making quality purchases: eatwellguide.org

Sprouting bulk items such as grains and legumes

Preparing food in bulk and freezing it to preserve nutrients

Obtaining nutrition from fresh foods to replace supplements

Using herbs and spices to enhance flavor

Eating seasonal food in greater variety (see Grocery List)

How to Sprout: Your Kitchen Garden

Why Sprout:

Sprouted foods are a unique nutrition source. Packed with protein, fiber, and minerals, sprouts deliver a combination of essential nutrients that show therapeutic benefits for managing a healthy body. These foods are your friends, and you bring them to life!

What You Can Sprout:

Dry seeds, grains, and legumes such as Lentils, mung beans, chia, pumpkin, buckwheat, quinoa and brown rice

Where to Find The Goods:

Bulk and "ethnic" sections in grocery store

Steps to Sprout (Growing Small Plants Indoors)

Keep out of direct sunlight for the entire process

1. Fill jar up 1/4 full with dry goods (1st timers use lentils)

2. Fill the rest of the jar with filtered water

3. Soak goods for 12 hours

4. Drain out water with a mesh screen

5. Rinse every 8 hours for 3-4 days (Do not refrigerate yet, this allows sprouts to grow)

6. Put goods in a container and refrigerate (sprouts last a week refrigerated)

Precautions for Sprouting

Bacteria can grow in a sprouting environment. Boiling the sprouts for 5 minutes kills most bacteria. Keeping these foods out of the sun, sterilizing the food environment with soap and hot water, rinsing sprouts frequently, and putting 1 tsp. of salt in with each rinse helps reduce bacteria.

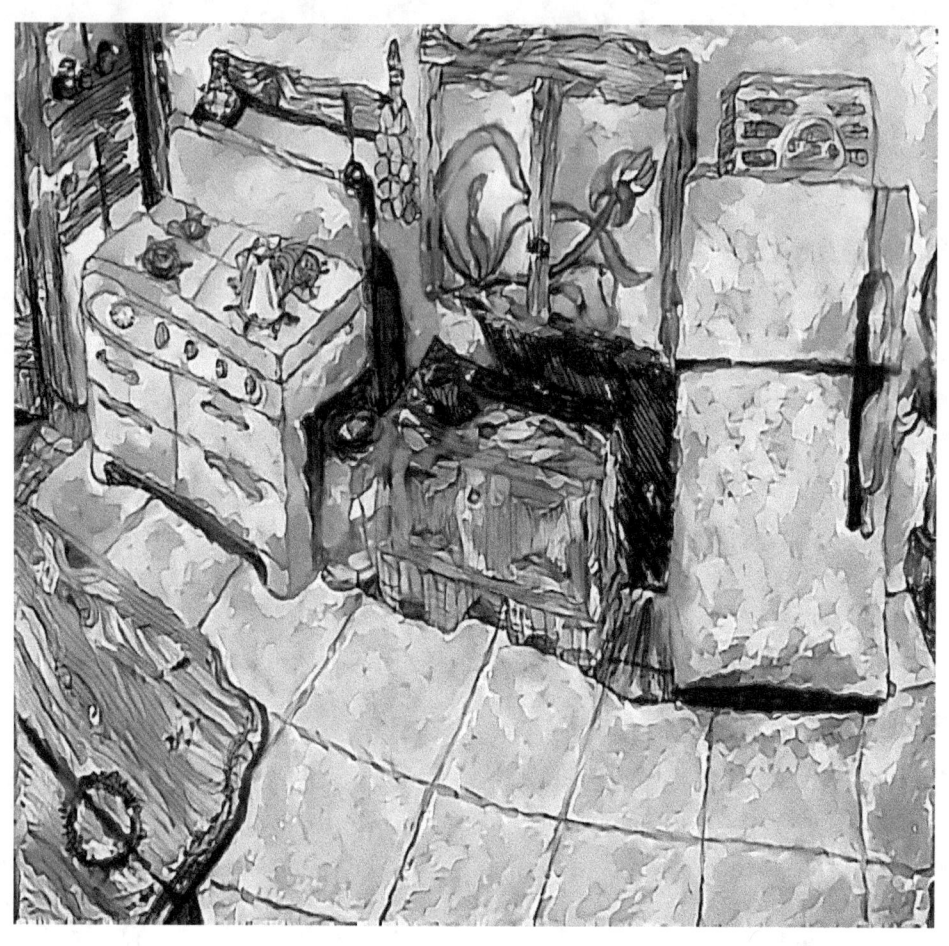

Useful Kitchen Tasks

Washing your hands:

Soap hands up to the wrists with warm water and rinse.

Shredding (aka Grating):

This task involves holding an item (carrot, beet, apple, zucchini, cucumber) to a "cheese grater" and grating that item to bits. This enhances flavor and juiciness.

Cracking eggs:

Tap egg lightly in the middle with a spoon, place thumbs on either side of the crack and pull the egg apart from this central crack.

Kitchenware:

Plates/bowls, utensils, natural soap, scrubber, towels, cups, blender, cheese grater, glass jars, large salad bowl and water filter.

Hand squeezed juice:

Slice orange/lemon in half with a knife. Put a fork into the middle of the half you are squeezing, and squeeze around the fork, with the open end of the fruit face down.

Knives:

Keep a lookout for fingers and toes. Always cut away from your body. Slice and dice to calming music please.

Spicing:

Less is more. Taste as you go. Stay stocked in salt, pepper, turmeric, garlic and cinnamon.

Making tea:

Once water boils, turn off heat, then add tea bags. Most teas only need to steep for 2-3 minutes to have the strongest flavor and active compounds.

Measuring conversions:

2.5 teaspoons (tsp.) = 1 tablespoon (TBS.)

16 tablespoons = 1 cup = 8 fluid ounces (oz)

2 cups = 1 pint

4 cups = 1 quart = 32 fluid ounces (oz)

16 cups = 1 gallon = 128 fluid ounces (oz)

Basic Vitality Grocery List

Green Vegetables
kale
chard
spinach
broccoli
asparagus
basil
lettuce
cilantro
parsley

Roots
carrot
beet
sweet potato
onion

Legumes
lentils
mung beans
chickpeas

Seeds
quinoa
hemp seed
chia seed
pumpkin seed

Spices
salt
pepper
garlic
turmeric
ginger
cinnamon

Fruit
apple
banana
berries
peach
pear
tomato

Citrus
lemon
lime
orange

Whole Grains
brown rice
amaranth
buckwheat

Animal Products
goat milk/cheese
sheep milk/cheese
eggs

Sauces
mustard
soy sauce
vinegar

Plant Fats
avocado
olive oil
coconut oil

List of Daily Staple Foods

For a 170 pound Male Athlete:

16 cups Filtered Water (1 cup per hour awake)

¼ cup Olive Oil/Coconut Oil

½ cup Hemp Seed

½ cup Chia Seed

½ cup Dry Buckwheat (sprouted – 72 hrs)

1 Avocado

2 Oranges

2 cups Dry Lentils (sprouted – 72 hrs)

10 Vegetables (5 cups)

2" Fresh Ginger Root

1 TBS. Sea Salt

Sun Dream
Sample Daily Tonic

Spice Tea:
1 TBS. Spirulina
1 tsp. Cinnamon
1 tsp. Turmeric
1 tsp. Ginger
1 tablet - Vitamin B12 1000 mcg

Mix all ingredients in a quart of warm water (add a teaspoon of honey for taste).

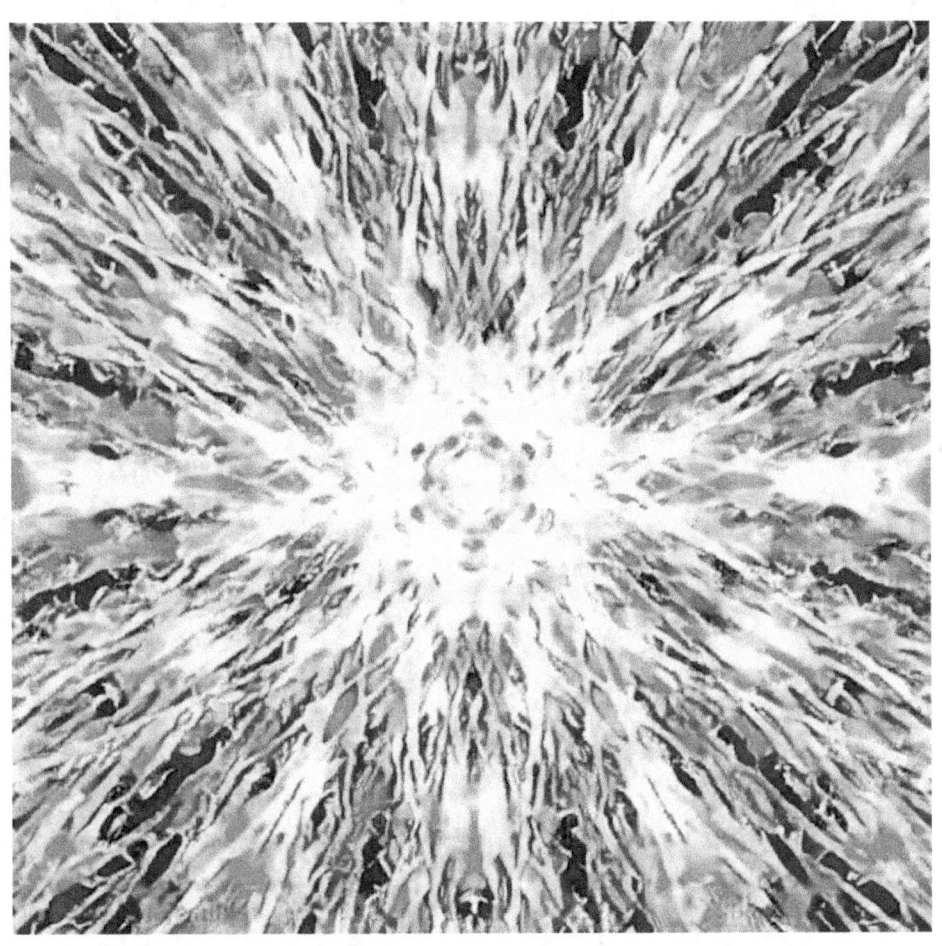

Camping Essentials

Characteristics: Long Shelf Life, Organic, Nutritious, Affordable, Calorically Dense, Lightweight

Non-Perishables (Good for Months)

Dry Grains/Legumes/Nuts/Seeds (see Simple Grocery Checklist)

Coconut Oil

Citrus

Salt

Dry Fruit/Honey

Spices and Teas

Native Edible Species (Wildcrafting)

Camping Essentials (continued)

Perishables (Good for One Week)

Roots (see Grocery Checklist)

Avocado

Kale

Fresh Fruit

Dehydrated Vegetarian Meals:
  harmonyhousefoods.com

Elements of Flavor

Fire : Ginger, Turmeric, Garlic, Pepper

Earth: Sage, Rosemary, Coriander, Cumin, Cinnamon

Wind: Mint, Basil, Parsley, Lavender, Oregano, Cilantro

Water: Citrus

Types of Tastes

Fresh, Crunchy, Chewy, Juicy, Crispy, Crisp, Tangy, Melty, Fluffy, Ruffled, Stringy, Pasty, Silky, Dense, Rich, Sweet, Sour, Bitter, Salty, Cheesy, Grainy, Starchy, Nutty, Creamy, Astringent, Fatty, Spicy, Acidic, Aromatic, Earthy, Pungent, Ambrosial

The Meal Crafting Process

Getting hungry!

Washing your hands.

Envisioning success.

Innovating every day.

Listening to appetizing music.

Making food with friends.

Following directions – amounts, times,

temperatures, order.

Cleaning as you go.

Watching your fingers.

Making an ideal dining atmosphere.

Sharing the moment.

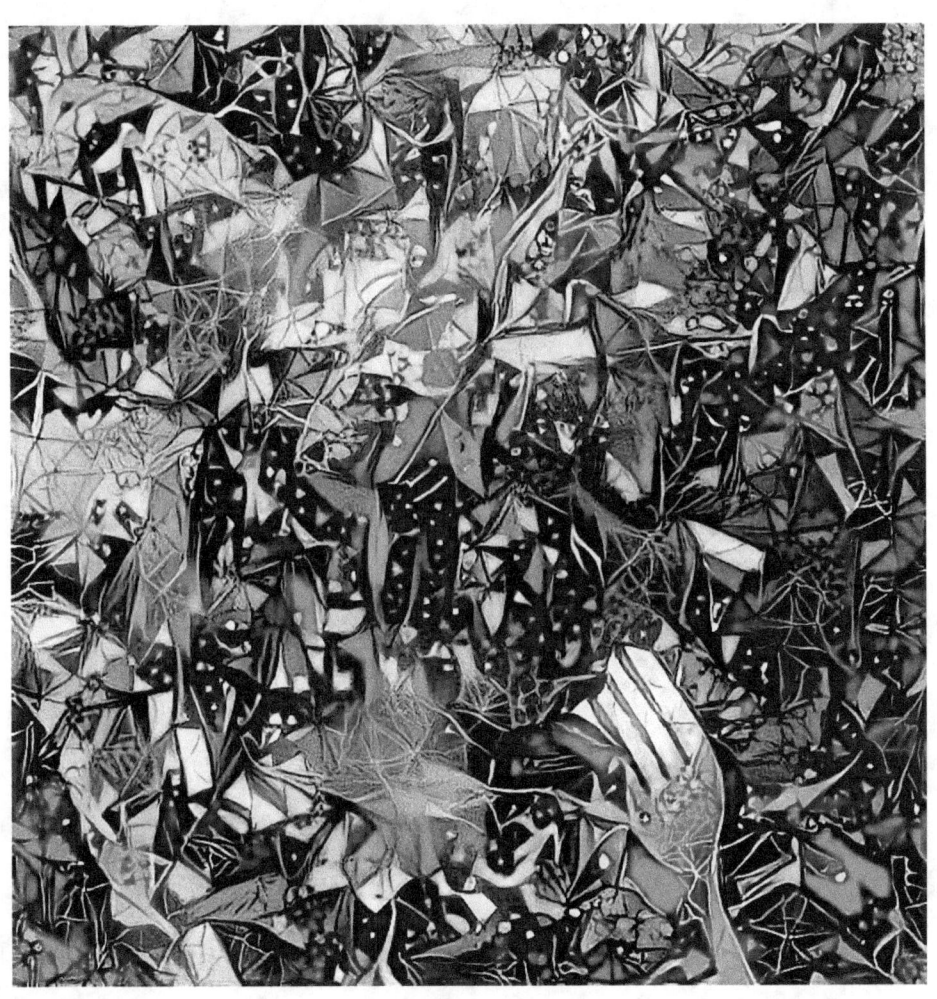

One-Step

Recipes

See "Medicinal Herbs" for a full list of
botanicals to power-up any of these meals.

Breakfast

Isakiate (Chia Tea)

Serves 2

Prep: 2 Minutes

½ cup Chia Seeds

4 cups Warm Water

1 Orange Juiced

Mix all ingredients in a large bottle.

Raw Granola Bar

Serves 2

Prep: 2 Minutes

1 cup Hemp Seeds

1 Apple (Chopped)

2 TBS. Sesame Seeds

1 TBS. Cinnamon

½ tsp. Nutmeg

2 TBS. Shredded Coconut (optional)

1/2 tsp. Salt

Mix all ingredients in a blender for 10 seconds, scoop into tupperware and compress the mixture with a spoon.

Fire Porridge

Serves 2

Prep: 10 Minutes

½ cup Hemp and/or Chia Seeds

2 TBS. Coconut Oil

½ cup Sprouted Buckwheat (optional)

½ cup Hot Water

1 TBS. Fresh Chopped Ginger

1 tsp. Cinnamon

1 tsp. Turmeric

½ cup Berries

Mix all ingredients in a bowl.

Earthy Scramble

Serves 2

Prep: 10 Minutes

6 Egg Whites

2 cups Chopped Kale

1/2 Red Onion (optional)

1 clove Chopped Garlic

¼ cup Chopped Cilantro

½ Avocado (topping)

1 tsp. Cumin

Salt and Pepper

Saute all ingredients in a pan.

GingerAid

Serves 2

Prep: 2 Minutes

1 cup Water

2 Oranges Juiced

1" Fresh Ginger Root

Mix all ingredients in a blender.

Avocado

Serves 1

Prep: 1 Minute

1 Avocado

Slice avocado in half, scoop it out with a spoon.

Entrée

All entrees can be made into soups, by blending all the ingredients and adding a cup of fresh water. This can help those with low digestive heat digest many of these high-fiber foods.

Purple Pumpkin

Serves 2

Prep: 5 Minutes

1 cup Raw Pumpkin Seeds

3 Shredded (grated) Carrots

1/2 Shredded (grated) Beet

1 TBS. Minced Garlic

1 TBS. Minced Ginger

¼ cup Chopped Cilantro

1 Avocado

2 TBS. Olive Oil

½ Orange Juiced

Mix all ingredients in a bowl.

Avocado Mash

Serves 2

Prep: 2 Minutes

1 Avocado or 2 TBS. Olive Oil

½ cup Hemp Seeds

½ Lemon juiced

Salt and Pepper

½ tsp. Cumin

¼ cup Chopped Cilantro

Mix all ingredients in a bowl.

Sprout Salad

Serves 2

Prep: 2 Minutes

3 cups Sprouted Mung Beans

1 cup chopped Dandelion Greens

½ cup Chopped Cilantro

1 Avocado

1 tsp. Oregano

1 tsp. Black Pepper

1 tsp. Sea salt

Mix all ingredients in a bowl.

Raw Cucumber Soup

Serves 4

Prep: 10 Minutes

2 cups Cucumber (chopped)

1 cup Zucchini (chopped)

1 Avocado (diced)

1 clove Garlic (chopped)

2 cups Water

1/2 Lemon Juiced

2 TBS. Olive Oil

Salt and pepper

Mix all ingredients in a blender.

Moroccan Spice Salad

Serves 4

Prep: 10 Minutes

6 Shredded (grated) Carrots

2 Shredded (grated) Beets

½ cup Raisins

2 TBS. Lemon Juice

2 TBS. Olive Oil

1 TBS. Honey

1 tsp. Cumin

1 tsp. Turmeric

1 tsp. Cinnamon

Salt and pepper

Mix all ingredients together in a large bowl.

Sushi Sprouts

Serves 2

Prep: 5 Minutes

3 cups Sprouted Mung Beans

½ cup Chopped Cilantro

1 Avocado

1 tsp. Oregano

1 tsp. Black Pepper

1 tsp. Coriander

1 tsp. Cumin

4 Sushi Wraps (Nori)

Mix all ingredients and wrap into the sushi.

Rawco (Raw Taco)

Serves 2

Prep: 5 Minutes

1 ear Sweet White Corn (Off the Cob)

1 Shredded (grated) Zucchini

1 Shredded (grated) Apple

3 Shredded (grated) Carrots

2 cups Chopped Dandelion

2 cups Sprouted Mung Beans

¼ cup Olive Oil

Salt and Pepper

6 Lettuce Leaves (the Taco Shells)

Mix all ingredients and scoop into the lettuce leafs.

Greenowa (Green Quinoa)

Serves 2

Prep: 5 minutes

1 cup Sprouted Quinoa

1 cup Sprouted Lentils

½ bunch Kale (chopped)

1 TBS. Oregano

2 TBS. Olive oil

1 TBS. Cilantro

1 clove Garlic

Simmer all ingredients in a pot for 5 minutes.

Fresh Rolls with Spicy Curry Sauce

Serves 2

Prep: 10 minutes

3 cups Baby Spinach

1 Zucchini (grated)

2 Carrots (grated)

3 leaves Red Cabbage (grated)

8 Rice Paper Rounds

Spicy Curry Sauce:

½ cup Cashews

1 Carrot (grated)

1 tsp. Turmeric

Wrap the vegetables in rice paper, and dip them into the Curry Sauce (blended).

Pesto Zucchini Pasta

Serves 2

Prep: 10 minutes

2 Zucchinis (grated)

2 Carrots (grated)

Pesto Sauce:

1/2 cup Walnuts

1/2 cup Pumpkin Seeds

1/2 cup Olive Oil

1 cup Fresh Basil

1/2 clove Garlic

Salt and pepper

Blend the pesto sauce and pour over your vegetable pasta.

Mango Summer Rolls

Serves 2

Prep: 10 minutes

8 sheets of Rice Paper

1 Mango (peeled and sliced)

1 Avocado (peeled and sliced)

1 Cucumber (grated)

½ cup Mint (chopped)

Spicy Almond Sauce:

1 TBS. Lime Juice

1 TBS. Ginger (minced)

1 TBS. Honey

¼ cup Almond Butter

Wrap the vegetables in rice paper, and dip them into the Spicy Almond Sauce (blended).

Macro Bowl

Serves 3

Prep: 10 minutes

1 head of Kale (chopped)

1 Carrot (grated)

1/2 cup Raw Sauerkraut

1/4 cup Hemp Seeds

1/2 cup Cherry Tomatoes

Garlic Basil Dressing:

½ Lemon Juiced

1 clove Garlic

1 cup Fresh Basil

¼ cup Water

Mix all ingredients in a bowl and pour on the Garlic Basil Dressing (blended).

Daikon Delectable

Serves 3

Prep: 10 minutes

1 Daikon Radish (grated)

1/4 cup Cucumber (chopped)

2 Carrots (grated)

2 TBS. Cilantro (chopped)

2 TBS. Raisins

Ginger Lime Dressing:

1 TBS. Honey

1 Lime Juiced

1 tsp. Ginger (grated)

2 TBS. Water

Mix all ingredients in a bowl and pour on the Ginger Lime Dressing (blended).

Lemon Curry Wild Rice

Serves 2

Prep: 10 minutes

1 cup Sprouted Wild Rice

1 Beet (grated)

1/4 cup Hemp Seeds

¼ cup Mint

Lemon Curry:

2 TBS. Olive Oil

1 TBS. Lemon Juiced

1 TBS. Ginger (sliced)

1 tsp. Coriander

1 tsp. Turmeric

Mix ingredients in a bowl and pour on the Lemon Curry.

Summer Fennel Salad

Serves 2

Prep: 10 minutes

1 bunch Dandelion Greens

1 cup Mung Bean Sprouts

2 TBS. Fresh Fennel

1 Cucumber (grated)

½ Avocado (diced)

1 Lime Juiced

2 TBS. Olive Oil

Salt and pepper

Mix all ingredients in a bowl.

Butternut Squash Soup

Serves 2

Prep: 2 Minutes

½ cup Water

½ cup Butternut Squash (chopped)

½ Cucumber (peeled)

1 TBS. Olive Oil

1" Fresh Ginger

1 tsp. Fresh Basil

Salt and pepper

Blend all ingredients.

Coconut Curry

Serves 4

Prep: 15 Minutes

3 cups Hot Water

1 cup Red Lentils

2 TBS. Coconut Oil

1 cup Coconut Milk

1 cup Shredded (grated) Carrot

1 cup Shredded (grated) Beet

2 cup Chopped Kale/Spinach/Dandelion

1 TBS. Fresh Cut Ginger

1 tsp. Turmeric

1 tsp. Black Pepper

1 tsp. Coriander

Simmer all ingredients in a pot for 10 minutes.

Lemon Ginger Stew

Serves 3

Prep: 5 Minutes

2 cups Hot Water

5 Carrots

5 Celery Stalks

1 Cucumber

1 Lemon Juiced

1 Avocado (optional)

1 TBS. Fresh Cut Ginger

1 tsp. Turmeric

1 tsp. Black Pepper

1 tsp. Cumin

Blend all ingredients in a blender, simmer on low heat for 5 minutes.

Sweet Kale

Serves 2

Prep: 10 Minutes

2 cup Chopped Kale

½ cup Hemp and/or Pumpkin Seeds

¼ cup Chopped Cilantro

1 Orange juiced

½ Avocado (topping)

Salt and Pepper

Saute kale in olive oil, then mix all ingredients in a bowl.

Curry Cauliflower Mash

Serves 4

Prep: 10 Minutes

1 Head of Cauliflower (chopped)

1 Cup Water

2 TBS. Olive Oil

2 Garlic Cloves

1 tsp. Turmeric

1" Fresh Chopped Ginger

1 tsp. Coriander

Salt and Pepper

Steam all ingredients in a pot on medium heat for 10 minutes, mashing cauliflower with a fork once it softens.

Broccoli Soup

Serves 4

Prep: 10 minutes

2 cups Water

1 bunch of Kale (chopped)

1 bunch of Broccoli (chopped)

1 Avocado (diced)

1 tsp. Turmeric

Salt and pepper

Simmer all ingredients in a pot for 10 minutes.

Coconut Tom Kha Sprouts

Serves 4

Prep: 10 minutes

4 cups Hot Water

1 cup Coconut Milk

1 TBS. Coconut Oil

1 bunch of Kale

4 cups Mung Bean Sprouts

1 tsp. Ginger

1 tsp. Garlic

1/2 tsp. Black Pepper

1/2 tsp. Coriander

½ tsp. Cumin

½ tsp. Nutmeg

Simmer all ingredients in a pot for 10 minutes.

Quinoa Tabouli Tacos

Serves 4

Prep: 10 minutes

2 cups Sprouted Quinoa

1 cup Parsley (chopped)

½ Onion (chopped)

4 Medium Shredded (grated) Carrots

1 Lime juiced

1 Cucumber (chopped)

2 Avocados (diced)

2 TBS. Olive Oil

2 TBS. Nutritional Yeast

Salt and pepper

8 Lettuce Leaves (Taco Shells)

Mix all ingredients and scoop into lettuce.

Hemp Nori Rolls

Serves 4

Prep: 10 Minutes

½ cup Hemp Seeds

1 cup Carrots (shredded)

1 TBS. Soy Sauce

1 clove Garlic (chopped)

1 tsp. Turmeric

1/2 cup Water

4 Nori sheets

Ground Mushrooms with Avo

Serves 4

Prep: 10 Minutes

¼ cup Pumpkin Seeds

1 cup Mushrooms

¼ cup Walnuts

½ White Onion (chopped)

2 TBS. Olive Oil

¼ cup Oregano

1 Avocado (chopped)

Salt and pepper

Blend all ingredients and top with avocado.

Garden Patties

Serves 4

Prep: 10 Minutes

1 cup Pumpkin Seeds

1 cup Hemp Seeds

4 Carrots (chopped)

1 Onion (chopped)

1 cup Parsley (chopped)

1 Lemon Juiced

3 tsp. Oregano

1 tsp. Turmeric

8 Lettuce Leaves (Buns)

Salt and pepper

Blend all ingredients and shape into patties, serve on lettuce leaves.

Green Burritos with Guac

Serves 4

Prep: 10 Minutes

4 Collard Green Leaves (Tortillas)

1 cup Mung Bean Sprouts

1 Cucumber (grated)

4 Carrots (grated)

Guacamole:

2 Avocados

½ Chopped White Onion

1 Chopped Tomato (optional)

½ cup Chopped Cilantro

1 Lemon or Lime juiced

1 tsp. Cumin

Wrap vegetables and guac into collard leaves.

Sauces

Guacamole

Serves 4

Prep: 5 Minutes

2 Avocados

½ Chopped White Onion

1 Chopped Tomato (optional)

½ cup Chopped Cilantro

1 Lime juiced

1 tsp. cumin

Salt and Pepper

Blend all ingredients together.

Lemon Curry Dressing

Serves 2

Prep: 5 Minutes

2 TBS. Olive Oil

1 TBS. Lemon Juiced

1 TBS. Ginger (sliced)

1 tsp. Turmeric

Salt and pepper

Blend all ingredients together.

Ginger Lime Dressing

Serves 2

Prep: 5 Minutes

1 Orange Juiced

1 Lime Juiced

1 tsp. Ginger (grated)

2 TBS. water

Blend all ingredients together.

Garlic Basil Dressing

Serves 2

Prep: 5 Minutes

½ Lemon

1 TBS. Tahini

1 clove Garlic

1 cup Fresh Basil

¼ cup Water

Blend all ingredients together.

Spicy Almond Sauce

Serves 2

Prep: 5 Minutes

1 TBS. Lime Juiced

1 TBS. Ginger (chopped)

1 clove Garlic (chopped)

1 TBS. Honey

2 TBS. Rice Vinegar

1 TBS. Olive Oil

¼ cup Almond Butter

Blend all ingredients together.

Pesto Sauce

Serves 2

Prep: 5 Minutes

1/2 cup Walnuts

1/2 cup Pumpkin Seeds

1/2 cup Olive Oil

1 cup Fresh Basil

1/2 clove Garlic

Salt and pepper

Blend all ingredients together.

Spicy Curry Sauce

Serves 2

Prep: 5 Minutes

½ cup Cashews

1 Carrot (grated)

1 Lemon Juiced

1 tsp. Cinnamon

1 tsp. Turmeric

1 tsp. Black Pepper

Blend all ingredients together.

Cheez Sauce

Serves 4

Prep: 5 Minutes

1 cup Cashews

1 Lemon Juiced

1/2 cup Water

2 TBS. Olive Oil

2 tsp. Oregano

4 TBS. Nutritional Yeast

Salt and pepper

Blend all ingredients together.

Rosemary Walnut Cheese

Serves 6

Prep: 10 Minutes

2 cups Walnuts

1 Probiotic Capsule

1/2 cup Water

2 TBS. Rosemary

Blend all ingredients, strain out excess water and store for 2 days *unrefrigerated* to ferment.

Zucchini Hummus

Serves 4

Prep: 5 Minutes

2 Zucchinis (chopped)

4 cloves Garlic

1/4 cup Olive Oil

1 Lemon Juiced

½ cup Pumpkin Seeds

Salt and pepper

Blend all ingredients together.

Dessert

Coconut Ice Cream

Serves 4

Prep: 5 minutes (+Freezing)

1 can of coconut milk

2 cups of any Fruit

2 TBS. Cinnamon (optional)

½ tsp. Vanilla

1 TBS. Sea Salt

Blend all ingredients together and freeze.

Carrot Cake

Serves 4

Prep: 5 minutes

4 Carrots (chopped)

1 cup Walnuts

1/2 cup Raisins

1 TBS. Cinnamon

Blend all ingredients.

Chocolate Fudge

Serves 4

Prep: 5 minutes

1 cup Walnuts

¼ cup Cacao or Carob

½ cup Coconut Oil

2 TBS. Honey

½ tsp. Vanilla

Blend all ingredients.

Elixirs

GingerAid

Serves 2

Prep: 2 Minutes

1 Cup Water

2 Oranges juiced

1" Fresh Ginger Root

Blend all ingredients.

NutMilk

Serves 4

Prep: 2 Minutes

3 cups Water

1 cup any Nuts or Seeds (soaked in water for 8 hrs prior)

1 TBS. Honey

¼ tsp. Vanilla

(add 1 TBS. Cinnamon to make "Horchata")

Blend all ingredients.

Blue Mango

Serves 4

Prep: 2 Minutes

1 cup Water

1 Mango (sliced)

1 cup Blueberries

½ tsp. Turmeric

Blend all ingredients.

Green Morning

Serves 4

Prep: 2 Minutes

1 cup Water

5 Celery Stalks (chopped)

1 Cucumber (peeled)

3 Carrots (chopped)

1 Lime Juiced

1" Fresh Ginger Root

Blend all ingredients.

Sun Tea

Serves 2

Prep: 3 Hours

4 cups Water

2 Bags any Tea (Loose Tea Leaves work too)

Place mixture in a large covered glass jar in direct sun for 3 hours.

Focus Tea

Serves 2

Prep: 5 Minutes

4 cups Water

2 TBS. Coconut Oil

2 Bags Green Tea

2 Bags Ginseng Tea

1 Lemon juiced

Boil water, add ingredients, let steep 5 min.

Muscle Tea

Serves 2

Prep: 5 Minutes

4 cups Water

2 TBS. Fresh Cut Ginger

1 tsp. Turmeric

1 Lemon juiced

Boil water, add ingredients, let steep 5 min.

Sleep Tea

Serves 2

Prep: 5 Minutes

4 cups Water

2 Bags Chamomile

1 Lemon juiced

1 tsp. Honey

Boil water, add ingredients, let steep 5 min.

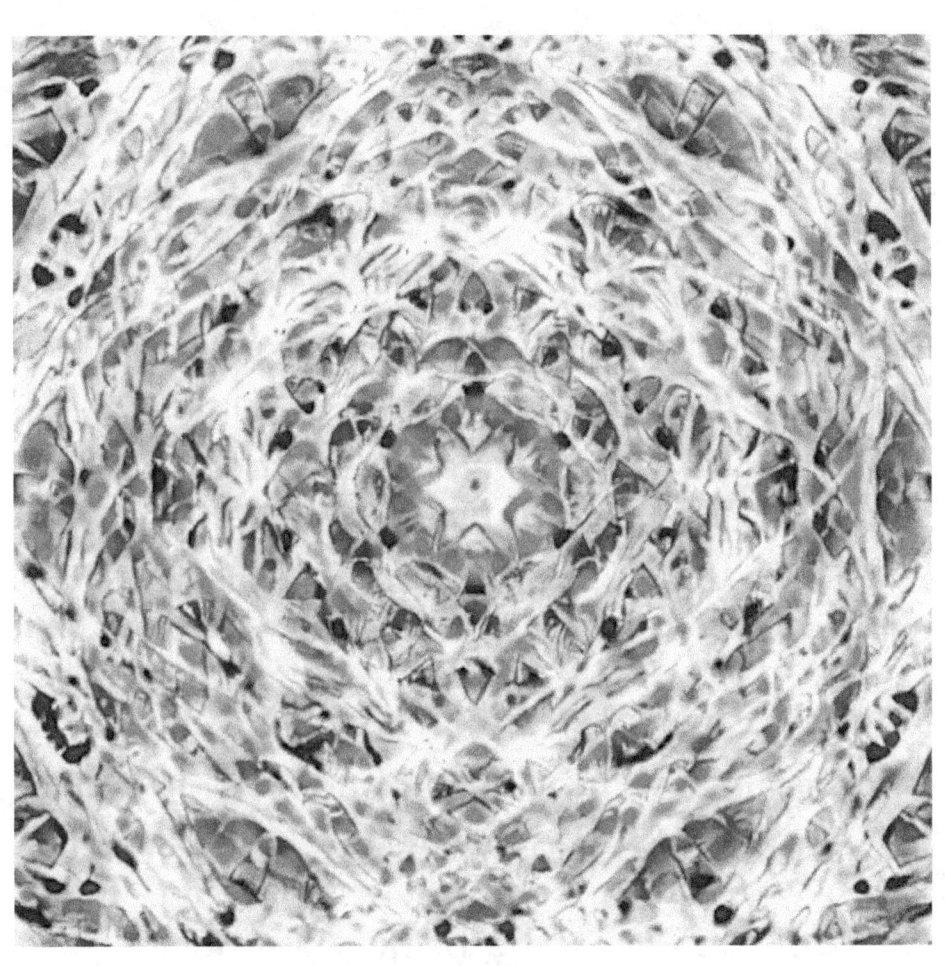

Medicinal Herbs and Uses

These plants stand the test of time as a part of the medical systems in China, India, Greece, Egypt and the Americas for thousands of years. All are regarded as safe for human consumption, with minimal side effects and interactions with other drugs. These herbs go by many names including: Tonic, Rasayana, Rejuvenative, Restorative, Adaptogen, Balancer, Stabilizer and Stress-Reliever. Imagine this list as millions of hours of trial and error condensed into one list.

As Stabilizers, these herbs help the body regulate homeostasis, so if something is too high, it gets lowered, and vice versa. All of these have antioxidant properties, essentially slowing the aging process and promoting vitality at all ages. As always, talk with a doctor and herbalist before medicating with these herbs especially if you have any medical conditions.

You can find organic versions of these items (in bulk) online. Cost per dose for each herb averages about 10 cents per day.

Blue-Green Algae (Spirulina and Chlorella)

Blue-Green Algae is commonly found in tropical and subtropical waters that contain a high salt content. It is used in boosting the immune system, improving memory, increasing energy (metabolism), lowering cholesterol, heart disease prevention, healing wounds, and improving digestion. Use caution with Autoimmune diseases and error on the side of of caution and avoid using if pregnant or breastfeeding.

Ginger Root

Ginger Root is native to warmer climates such as China, Japan, India, South America, Africa, and Middle East. It is used to treat stomach problems related to motion sickness, gas, diarrhea, irritable bowel, nausea, arthritis, osteoarthritis, menstrual pain, migraines, bronchitis, and diabetes. Using ginger root may cause increased risk of bleeding with someone with bleeding disorders, cause increased insulin levels and/or lower blood sugar.

Turmeric Root

Turmeric Root originates from Southern India and derived from the Turmeric Plant. Used to treat arthritis, heartburn, joint pain, stomach pain, Crohn's disease, ulcerative colitis, diarrhea, stomach bloating, loss of appetite, jaundice, liver problems, irritable bowel syndrome, gallbladder disorders, high cholesterol, skin inflammation, bronchitis, colds, and lung infections. May slow blood clotting, cause upset stomach, and decrease blood sugar in people with diabetes.

Parsley, Dandelion and Cilantro

Is found natively in China and Mexico. Used to treat digestion problems, loss of appetite, hernia, nausea, diarrhea, bowel spasms, intestinal gas, hemorrhoids, toothaches, and joint pain. May consider avoiding any dosage if pregnant.

Ceylon Cinnamon Bark

Ceylon Cinnamon is from the inner bark of several trees from the genus Cinnamomum. Used to treat gastrointestinal upset, menstrual cramps, colds, and the flu. Can lower blood sugar with type 2 diabetes.

Red Reishi Mushroom

Red Reishi Mushrooms are found in China and Korea. It is used for boosting the immune system, viral infections, swine flu, avian flu, lung conditions (asthma and bronchitis), heart disease, kidney disease, cancer, liver disease, HIV, altitude sickness, chronic fatigue, insomnia, stomach ulcers, poisoning, and herpes pain. May cause increased bleeding and may lower blood pressure.

Ginseng Root

This root is found in Siberia, Asia, and the Americas. It can be used for stress, boost the immune system, and gastritis. Avoid using if pregnant, may lower blood sugar with people with diabetes, causes sleep problems and agitation for mental conditions.

Astragalus Root

Found in China, Mongolia and North Korea. It is used to treat common cold, upper respiratory infections, allergies, fibromyalgia, anemia, HIV, chronic fatigue syndrome, kidney disease, diabetes, and high blood pressure. Avoid using if have you have an Autoimmune Disease, due to Astragalus can make the immune system more active.

Schisandra Berry

Found mainly in China and Russia. Used to prevent early aging, normalizing blood sugar, blood pressure, stimulating the immune system, treating liver disease, high cholesterol, coughs, asthma, insomnia, spontaneous sweating, involuntary discharge of semen, erectile dysfunction, exhaustion, excessive urination, depression, irritability, and memory loss. Side effects include increased stomach acid with individuals that have GERD disease.

Moringa Leaf

Native to the Africa and sub-Himalayan areas of India, Pakistan, Bangladesh, and Afghanistan. Moringa can be used for anemia, arthritis, rheumatism, asthma, cancer, constipation, diabetes, diarrhea, epilepsy, stomach pain, stomach and intestinal ulcers, intestinal spasms, headache, heart problems, high blood pressure, kidney stones, fluid retention, thyroid disorders, and infections. Avoid using if pregnant due to the chemicals in the root, bark, and flowers can make the uterus contract, and this might cause a miscarriage.

Tulsi Leaf (Holy Basil)

Originally from India, it stills grows in most gardens there. Used to treat colds, flus, H1N1 flu, diabetes, bronchitis, earache, headache, stomach upset, heart disease, fever, viral hepatitis, stress, and tuberculosis. Side effects encountered is slow blood clotting.

Suma Root

Is a ground vine plant found in South America. Suma Root is used to treat cancer and tumors, diabetes, male sexual performance problems, and applied to the skin for wounds and skin problems. Suma can cause asthma symptoms if the root powder is inhaled.

Licorice Root

Licorice Root is the root of Glycyrrhiza glabra native to southern Europe and parts of Asia, such as India. Used to treat stomach ulcers, bronchitis, osteoarthritis, lupus, malaria, tuberculosis, and CFS. When used for several weeks it can cause high blood pressure, low potassium levels, weakness, paralysis, and occasionally brain damage.

Gotu Kola Leaf

It is a small, herbaceous plant and is native to wetlands in Asia. Used to treat infections, shingles, leprosy, cholera, dysentery, syphilis, colds, flu, H1N1, tuberculosis, and schistosomiasis. May cause too much sleepiness if combined with medications used during and after surgery.

Brahmi Leaf

An herb native to the wetlands of Asia, Africa, Europe, and South America. Brahmi is used for Alzheimer's, improving memory, anxiety, ADHD, backache, mental illness, epilepsy, and joint pain. Side Effects include increased secretions in urinary tract, may cause increased levels of thyroid hormone, could worsen lung conditions (Asthma), slow down heart beat, and cause congestion in intestines.

Osha Root

Grows above 7,000 feet throughout the entire Rocky Mountain Range from Mexico to Canada. Used to treat sore throats, bronchitis, cough, colds, influenza, swine flu, viral infections, and pneumonia. Side effects are menstruation and may cause miscarriages.

Shilajit Mineral Pitch

Is found predominantly in the Himalaya mountains of Asia, it is millions of year old plant matter squeezed out of cracks in the rocks by tectonic plate movement. Used to treat arthritis, stress, and aging (both mental and physical). Side effects are lower blood pressure and adversely affect diabetics for the same reason.

Cannabis Leaf

It is found in Africa, Eurasia and the Americas. Used as a sedative, muscle relaxant and euphoriant that can relieve some side effects of drugs and can help patients to live through serious illnesses. Side effects are depersonalization and acute anxiety.

Oregano Leaf Oil

It is native to temperate western and southwestern Eurasia and the Mediterranean region. Oregano Leaf oil is taken by mouth to treat intestinal parasites, allergies, sinus pain, arthritis, cold and flu. It is also applied to the skin to treat acne, athlete's foot, dandruff, canker sores, warts, ringworm, rosacea, and psoriasis. Sides effects that it may cause are increased risk of bleeding, allergic reaction, and low blood sugar.

Black Cumin Seed Oil

Is native to the Mediterranean and Middle East. Used to treat MRSA infection, epilepsy, heavy metal poisoning, tumors, diarrhea, increase urine flow, menstruation. Black Cumin is known to slow blood clotting and lower blood sugar.

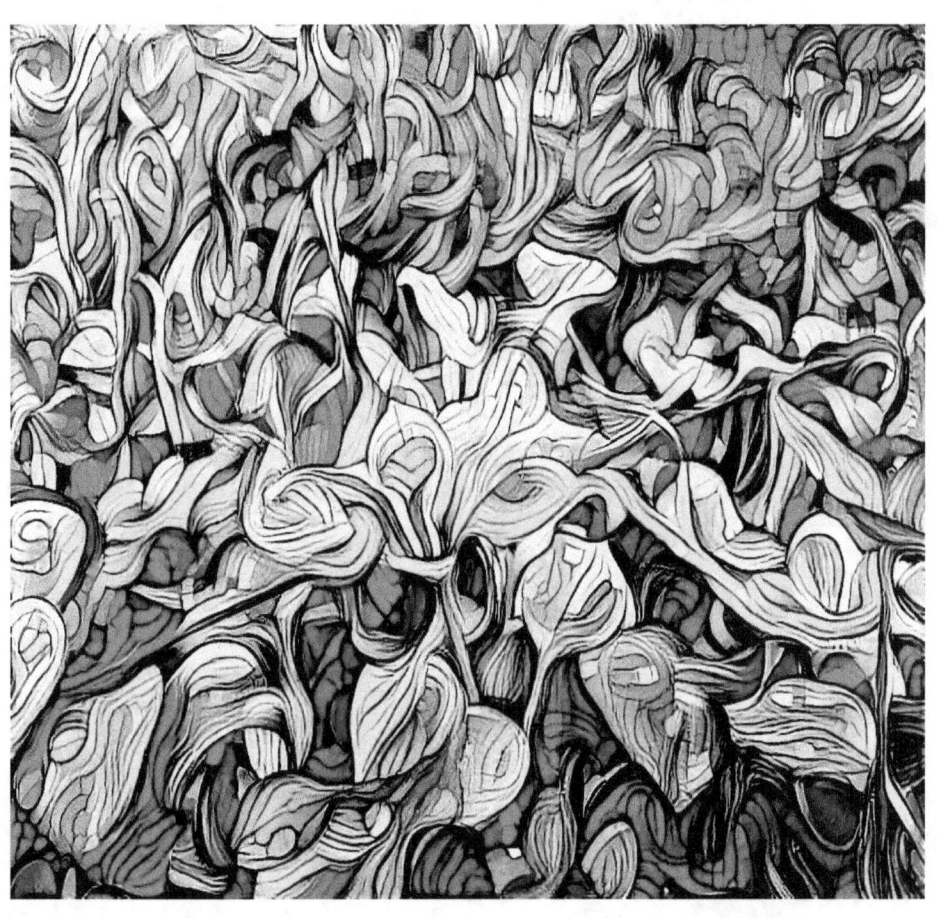

Three

Natural Science

Living Food and The Nanotechnology of You

All animals, besides humans (and dumpster-diving racoons), eat only raw food. In the scope of evolutionary time, cooking foods is a recent phenomenon, along with writing. Such strategies allow us to communicate to one another new ways of perceiving the world through our sensory organs, providing stimulation, which spurs the learning process.

Raw plants do the digestive work for you by providing essential enzymes your body otherwise has to make. Enzymes are nature's nanotechnology, allowing you to think and live life, while these intelligent plant machines restore the genetic structure of your body.

Digestive plant enzymes remain intact below 115° F. Cooking foods destroys these delicate plant enzymes, and the bioavailability of water-soluble antioxidants (vitamins) in cooked food is, on average, 50% fewer than raw. Nutrients in cooked foods include fats and fat-soluble minerals, carbohydrates and proteins.

Raw Food = Less Digestive Work = More Energy

By eating foods in the state that they grow, you give your body the opportunity to connect to a system that operates on the wisdom of ecological communication. Through this process of interaction, the body can restore itself. Raw foods detoxify the body, and since toxins are stored in fat, fat melts away with minimal effort.

The Principles of Nature

Nature runs on sunlight

Nature uses only the energy it needs

Nature fits form to function

Nature recycles everything

Nature rewards collaboration

Nature requires diversity

Nature demands local expertise

Nature curbs excesses from within

Nature knows the power of limits

-Naturalist J. M. Benyus

Being in a Happy Body

Requirement: Being happy for what's here, your body, your family, air to breathe, time to think, ability to speak.

"I am hopelessly and forever a mountaineer, and I care only to entice people to look at Nature's loveliness." - John Muir

Wherever you are on your quest for knowledge, you can find peace in knowing that your body is encoded with many millions of years of genetic information to keep the internal computer of your "user experience" running smoothly. The phrase, "If it ain't broke, don't fix it!" applies to daily living and species evolution. Any imbalance you have and feel are messages from your body system to take care of yourself and pay close attention to where you are and what you are doing. You can adapt to adversity in infinite ways.

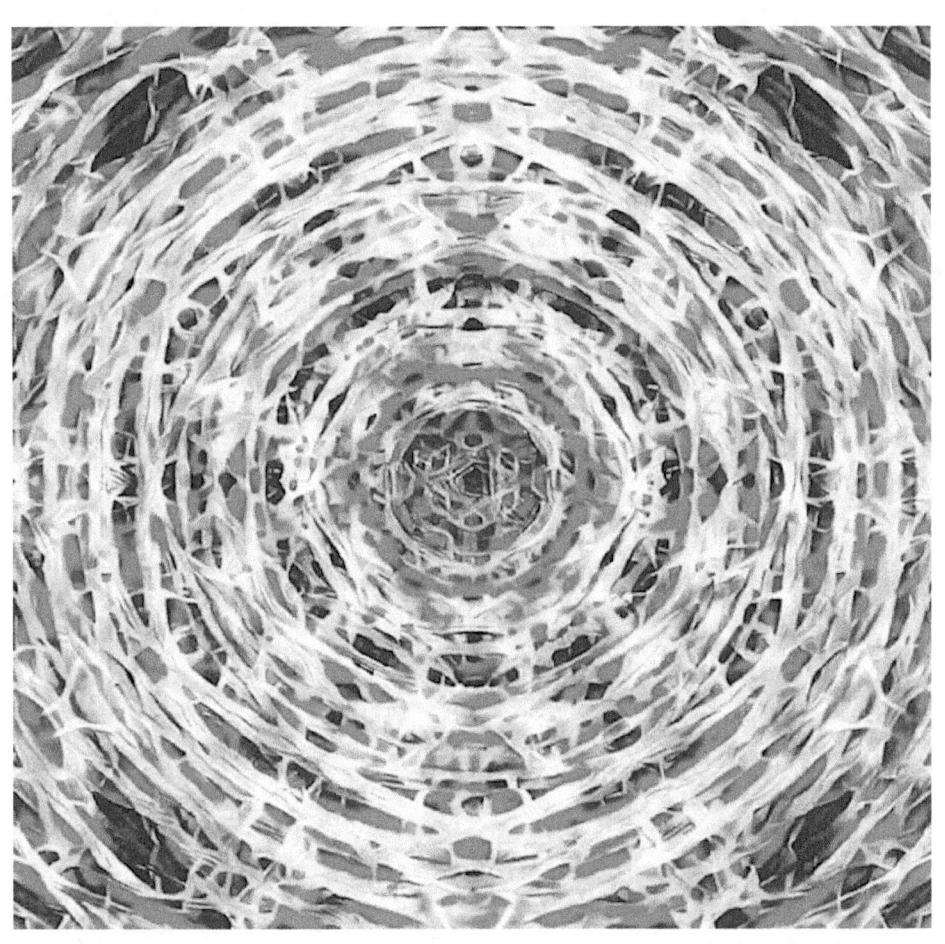

Body Maintenance Essentials

Maintain a tranquil mind
Sit still like a tortoise
Walk sprightly like a pigeon
Sleep like a dog

Tips for Body Maintenance

Rule #1: Your body knows best

Applying dogmatic principles can help manage health (i.e. avoiding all animal products)

If you struggle with following *dogmatic principles*, you can *create value* based on that principle (Dogma: never eating meat / Value: living with respect for all life)

Clean food, clean place, clean face

Knowing where your food comes from helps you know where you come from

Food from a happy home helps you live in a happy home

Savoring each bite - "Drink your food, chew your water"

You eat best when you are hungry

Body Maintenance (continued)

You can reflect on willpower to understand it

Eating a light protein before exercise improves performance (chia seeds)

Ginger and turmeric help restore muscle tone and detoxify entire system

Fasting one day per week improves metabolism

Restricting caloric intake increases longevity

Fat (2 TBS nuts/coconut oil) before bed relieves insomnia

Vegetables digest well with all foods, protein and carbohydrates do best separate

Body Maintenance (continued)

Choosing 3 meals for each mealtime that you can master and enjoy, including one meal that you prepare and bring with you on the day's adventure (see Recipes)

Waking up to 32oz water with a lemon alkalizes body pH and hydrates all cells

Drinking water away from mealtimes helps digestion

Refrigerated leftovers are best used within 24 hours to preserve vital energy

Sun-cooking/steaming food preserves nutrients and soften the fibers

Using only the leaves (and composting the stalk) of green vegetables reduces fiber

Meals with 3 main ingredients + seasonings keep your digestive system relaxed

Body Maintenance (continued)

Preparing meals in bulk in advance saves time, you can freeze leftover

Your body requires 50 essential nutrients to produce over 50,000 compounds

You can find all 50 essential nutrients in plants – except vitamin B12, which comes from a bacteria in soil and very few plants (spirulina and chlorella algae, moringa tree, nori seaweed) - supplement with a B12 tablet

Going to bed hungry improves protein metabolism

Protein and fat reduce sugar craving, fruit (sugar) causes insulin spike promoting fat gain (green vegetables provide all vitamins found in fruit)

"Ceylon Cinnamon" balances blood sugar (for therapeutic dose 2 tsp. 2x a day)

Body Maintenance (continued)

Cooking food preserves minerals, reduces vitamins/enzymes, and softens fibers

Raw plant foods contain essential live enzymes that protect your body

Tracking your daily habits allows you to observe change.

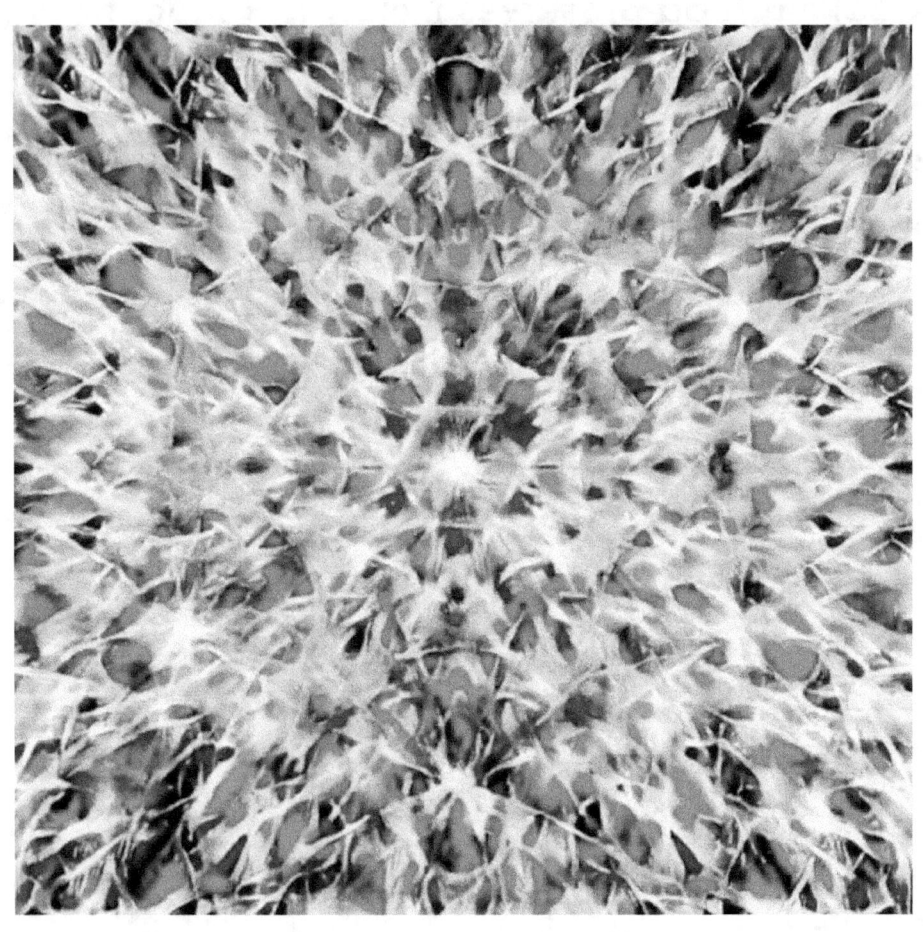

"The greatest fear in the world is of the opinions of others, and the moment you are unafraid of the crowd, you are no longer a sheep, you become a lion. A great roar arises in your heart, the roar of freedom." - Osho

The Immune System: Autoimmunity

"Autoimmunity" happens when the body creates an abnormal immune response against itself. This covers a range of experiences (physical conditions) we commonly call disease. The medical community shows a genetic similarity between all of these conditions, and for the most part, these conditions are triggered by inflammation.

Correlated genetic "triggers" for inflammation:
Physical and emotional stress (Fear)
Food allergens (Dietary Lectin)
Environmental Toxins (Pathogens and
　　Chemicals in Synthetic Food/Cosmetic
　　Products)

Common Autoimmune (Inflammatory) Conditions

Thyroiditis
Multiple Sclerosis
Fibromyalgia
Lupus
Celiac Disease
Rheumatoid Arthritis
Psoriasis
Scleroderma
Meniere's Disease

Inflammation is the body's natural response to heal damaged cells caused by bacteria, pathogens, allergens, and injuries. The body sends fresh oxygenated blood to the injured region, which usually produces swelling, stiffness and pain. One can begin to manage any inflammatory condition with the following recommendations.

The next section is for helping a person with autoimmunity (what we call a "chronic" condition). While the following recommendations are far from the sum of the medical literature, this does not constitute as medical advice.

Please, only attempt to follow these recommendations under the guidance of a trained medical professional. Everyone heals differently – these are steps to improve muscle, bones, blood, and overall physical quality.

How to Manage Autoimmunity

Alleviating Disease by Restoring Proper Digestion

1. Ask a Physician to test you for:
    Infections – yeast, bacteria, virus (notably Candida and H. Pylori)
    Food allergies with an IgG test.
    Heavy metal toxicity. (Raw Parsley is one of the most effective plants for removing heavy metals from the body)
    TNF-Alpha levels via adiponectin. (avoid foods high in Lectin enzyme)
2. Exercise regularly.
3. Practice relaxation techniques (nature walks, yoga, deep breathing, biofeedback, massage)
4. Eat organic food – 10 raw vegetables a day (blenders help) (avoid dietary Lectin)
5. Avoid consuming canola/sunflower oils, refined sugars, alcohol and grains (as well as

environmental toxins in processed/GMO food, cosmetics, and plastic bottles)

6. Drink pure water. (tap water often contains heavy metals)

7. Have a doctor recommend herbal adaptogens for digestion, inflammation and relaxation (Turmeric, Spirulina/blue-green algae, Guggul, Ginger, Reishi).

8. Get a second, third and fourth opinion after your MD/endocrinologist - from an Ayurvedic Physician, Yoga Teacher/Personal Athletic Trainer and a Naturopathic Doctor/Functional Medicine MD.

functionalmedicine.org/practitioner

Autoimmune (Alkalizing) List

All Vegetables (with two exceptions)

artichoke, arugula, asparagus, bamboo, broccoli, brussels sprout, cabbage, cauliflower, celery, cilantro, chard, collard greens, cucumber, fennel, green bean, kale, leek, lettuce, parsley, pumpkin, rhubarb, spinach, squash, watercress

Avoid nightshades: tomatoes, white potato, eggplant and peppers

Be sure to fully cook crucifers such as kale, spinach, cabbage, broccoli and cauliflower

Autoimmune (Alkalizing) List

Fruit (with two exceptions)

apple, apricot, avocado, banana, berries,
cherry, coconut, date, fig, grape, grapefruit,
guava, kiwi, lemon, lime, mango, nectarine,
orange, papaya, peach, pear, persimmon,
plum, pineapple, pomegranate, tangerine

Avoid Melons

*Fruit sugar (fructose) increases fat storage,
    which can produce inflammation — limit to 3
    fruits (1 cup) per day*

Herbs

basil, bay leaf, chamomile, chives, dill,
lavender, lemongrass, marjoram, mint,
oregano, parsley, peppermint, rosemary,
sage, spearmint, tarragon, thyme

Autoimmune (Alkalizing) List

Roots

beet, carrot, ginger, jicama, onion, parsnip, turnip, radish, rutabaga, shallot, sweet potato, turmeric, yam

Animals (with two exceptions)

land animals, fish, shellfish, insects!

Avoid processed meat (factory farmed)

One can gain all essential nutrients from plant foods

Spices

anise, cinnamon, cloves, garlic, ginger, saffron, shallots, turmeric

Fats and Oils

coconut, olive, avocado

Autoimmune (Alkalizing) List

Physicians recommend that people with autoimmunity avoid certain food groups including certain fats, dairy, eggs, and anything that has a "seed husk" or shell, such as grains, seeds and nuts.

Some individuals with autoimmunity report that after soaking and sprouting foods with a seed husk, these foods are better digested.

A rule of thumb is that the smaller grains, legumes and seeds are easier to digest.

Everyone is different. These foods are included as Frontier Foods to experiment.

Autoimmune Frontier Foods (Special Consideration)

* Soaked and Sprouted Grains: such as Oats, Rice and Buckwheat

Eliminate Gluten (Wheat) Foods

* Soaked and Sprouted Legumes: such as Beans and Nuts

Avoid Peanuts and Soybeans

* Soaked and Sprouted Seeds: such as Hemp, Chia, Pumpkin, Flax, Sesame, Sunflower, Quinoa

Autoimmune (Alkalizing) List

Foods to Avoid

Physicians generally recognize these foods and products as triggers for Autoimmunity and Inflammation.

*Grains: such as Oats, Rice, Wheat (*Eliminate* Gluten)

*Seeds: such as Flax, Sunflower, Quinoa and others

*Legumes: such as Beans, Nuts, Soybeans

Cow Dairy Products: Cheese, Yogurt, Butter, Ice Cream, Milk

Eggs

Nightshades: Tomatoes, White Potato, Eggplant and All Peppers

Autoimmune (Alkalizing) List Foods to Avoid (continued)

Refined Sugars: Sugar, corn syrup, coconut sugar – limit maple syrup and honey

Alcohol: (substitute with Kombucha and Herbal Tea)

Food Additives: carageenan, guar gum, aspartame, MSG, sulfates/sulfites, nitrates/nitrites, magnesium stearate

NSAIDs: Ibuprofin (Advil), Naproxen, and others (these are technically called "anti-inflammatory drugs" that trigger autoimmunity – substitute with White Willow Bark and Turmeric)

Personal Considerations

Age: You eat more when you're young and hungry.

Activity: Eating better = doing more = feels like doing less.

Blood type: A, B, AB, O, Rh-

Genetics: Eating food that grows in your ancestral geography.

Goals: Athletic, Cosmetic, Medicinal, Religious, Survival

Budget: Time, Money, Energy

Location Access: Urban, Agrarian, Desert, Jungle

Culture: Varies from home to home, city to city, state to state, country to country

Specific Protocols

Omnivorous

Pescatarian

Fruitarian

Vegetarian

Vegan

Raw

Paleolithic

Blood-Type

Ayurvedic

Macrobiotic

Autoimmune

Anti-Inflammatory

Home-Grown

Allergen-Free

Low-Glycemic

Ketogenic

Plant-Based

Non-GMO

Local

Organic

Seven Survival Foods

And Relevant Macro and Micronutrients

Green Leaves: Protein, Vitamin A, C, E, & K,
  Iron, Calcium, Zinc, Magnesium
Sprouts: Protein, Vitamin C, Carbohydrates,
  Iron, Potassium
Seeds (Hemp, Pumpkin and Chia): Protein,
  Omega-3 Fat
Avocado: Protein, Omega-3 Fat
Citrus (Lemon, Lime and Orange): Vitamin C
Turmeric: Curcumin
Garlic: Allicin

The "Survival" Quality

You can live well on these foods alone.

In total, they provide the essential nutrients in
addition to "non-essential" compounds that
support a vibrant life (aka you can live on
these foods) and you can mix them all
together for a hearty meal.

Available in an unprocessed, natural state
Promoting Digestive Fire
Anti-Inflammatory
Antioxidant Rich
Body Alkalizing
Cost Effective
Allergen-Free
Humane
Simple
Tasty

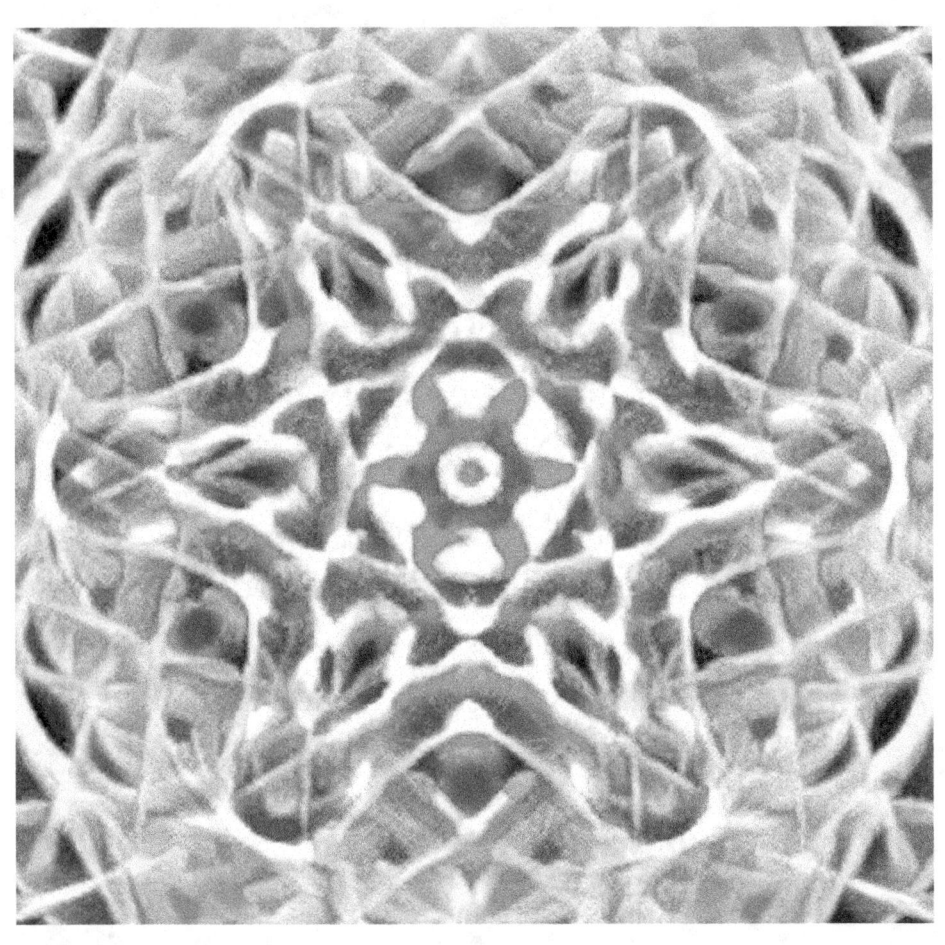

Essential Nutrients: Functional Foods

<u>Clean Water</u> = Fresh Filtered Water

<u>Macronutrients</u>

Protein (Amino Acids) – Body Rebuilding

sprouted beans, seeds and whole grains

Fat (Free Fatty Acids) – Muscle/Joint/Organ Tissue Mobility

avocado, hemp/flax/chia seeds, coconut

Carbohydrates (Glucose) – Body Fuel

sprouted beans and whole grains, roots

Fiber (Technically Carbohydrate) – Digestion

most plant foods

Micronutrients

Vitamins (Antioxidants and Enzymes)

Minerals

Bacteria (Pre- and Pro-biotics)

Water: The Freshest of All

Water is fresh. Water is life. Therefore, fresh is life. Taste a sip of water to know what you are made of. Listen to water to and see its effects all around you, in a cloud, in the rain, in a river, in the sea, on a mountain peak. Feel it, flow it.

Protein: Rebuilding the Body

The term protein refers to 20 enzymes (the 20 amino acids – 9 essential, 11 non-essential) which undergo a series of reactions to be used in every cell in the body. All food contains protein, with different proportions of amino acids, and the type and quality differ dramatically. For example, spinach has a similar amino acid profile to chicken, and one chicken leg has equal protein amount (15g) to 5 cups of spinach. Remember Popeye the Sailor Man.

For those who use plants for protein, the most important amino acid to take into consideration is lysine. It's important to iterate that all foods are complete proteins (containing all amino acids *in different proportions*). Animal products contain relatively higher amounts of lysine than plants, with the few exceptions listed here.

Plant Sources of Lysine

1. Pistachios and pumpkin seeds

2. Mung beans

3. Lentils

Note: Soy products and fermented wheat (tofu/tempeh/seitan) are technically the highest plant-food sources of lysine, excluded from this list due to heavy processing and the subsequent effects on hormone regulation.

Plant Protein List

(Measured in Grams)

Nut/Seed (1/4 Cup; 4 tbs)

Chia Seed 12
Hemp Seed 12
Flax Seed 8
Sunflower Seed 8
Salba 7
Almond 7
Pumpkin Seed 7
Sesame Seed 7
Pistachio 6
Walnut 5
Brazil Nut 5
Hazelnut 5
Cashew 4
Avocado*, 1 medium, 4 (*yes, it's a fruit)

Beans (1 Cup sprouted)

Lentil 18
Adzuki 17
Cannellini (white beans) 17
Navy Bean 16
Split Peas 16
Anasazi 15
Black Bean 15
Garbanzos (chick peas) 15
Kidney Bean 15
Mung Beans 14
Pinto Beans 14
Green Peas 9

Grains (1 Cup sprouted)

Millet 8
Amaranth 7
Oat Bran 7
Wild Rice 7
Buckwheat 6
Barley 5
Quinoa 5
Brown Rice 5

Vegetables

Corn, 1 large cob, 5
Collard Greens, 1 cup, 4
Artichoke, medium, 4
Broccoli, 1 cup, 4
Mushrooms, 1 cup, 4
Swiss Chard, 1 cup, 3
Kale, 1 cup, 3
Asparagus, 5 spears, 2
String Beans, 1 cup, 2
Beets, 1 cup, 2
Sweet Potato, 1 cup, 3
Cabbage, 1 cup, 2
Carrot, 1 cup, 2
Cauliflower, 1 cup, 2
Celery, 1 cup, 1
Spinach, 1 cup, 1
Cucumber, 1 cup, 1
Leeks, 1 cup, 1
Lettuce, 1 cup, 1

Fat: Fueling the Furnace

The brain is 60% fat, which insulates the wiring of your nervous system to help your body move, reason and love (and stay warm). Most vitamins bind to fat in order for us to digest them. The body readily converts healthy fats (avocado, olive oil, seeds) into energy (glucose) through "gluconeogenesis." This process allows the body to burn fat for fuel and conserve carbohydrates and protein as reserve energy sources. Three pounds of body fat represents 10,000 calories - how much an average climber burns in a day trekking up Mount Everest. In general, eating healthy fat helps your body get used to burning fat and melts away accumulated body fat.

Omega Rich Fats

Avocado

Walnuts

Pumpkin Seeds

Chia Seeds

Hemp Seeds

Coconut Oil

Olive Oil

Carbohydrates: Photosynthetic Energy

Carbohydrate (glucose) is the direct product of photosynthesis, and a form of microscopic "currency" in the economy of organic lifeforms such as plants, bacteria, and fungi. Bacteria transform proteins and micronutrients that fungi decompose to a useable form, and trade those minerals for excess carbohydrates. We then, eat plants (and occasionally fungi and some dirt) and gain carbohydrates (in addition to protein and minerals provided by bacteria) from the plants, and use that as a fuel source for each day under the sun. Carbohydrates provide readily useable energy for us to stay active.

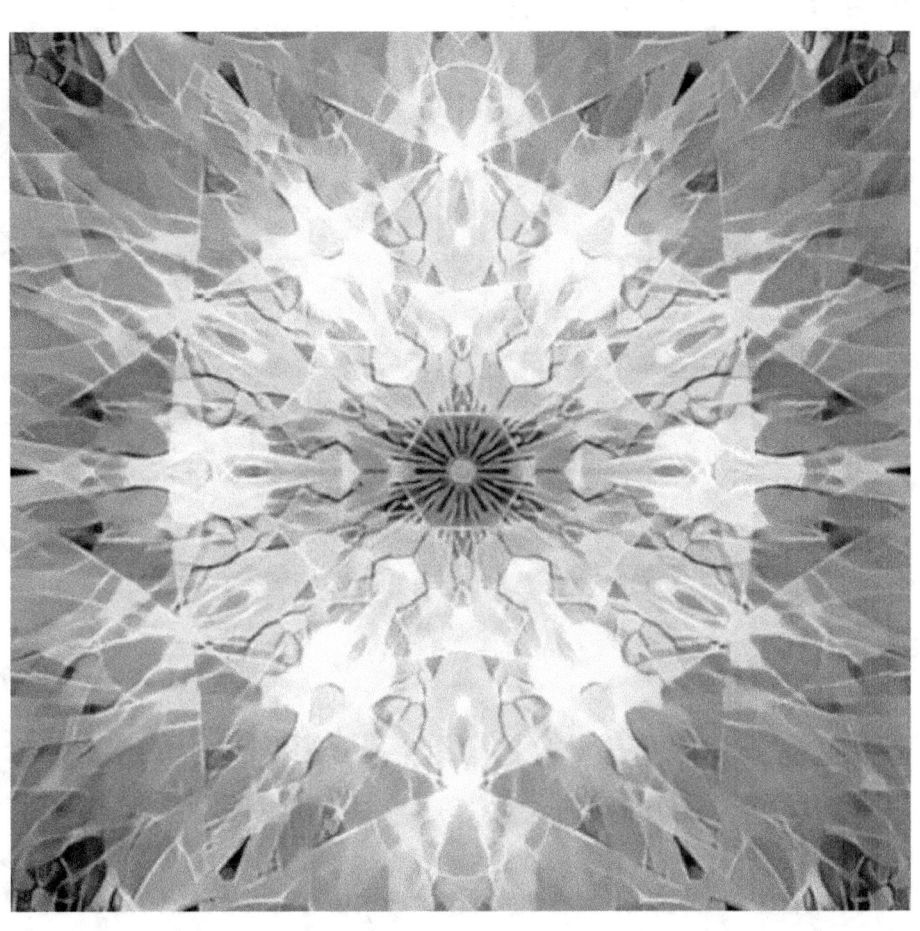

Vitamins

Essential Antioxidants

Vitamin A – Vision Health (leafy greens, carrots, sweet potatoes)

B Vitamins – Brain Function

(green vegetables, sprouted legumes/seeds/whole grains) *Supplement Vitamin B_{12}*

Vitamin C – Cell Recovery (<u>raw</u> vegetables and fruits)

Vitamin D – Muscle/Joint/Organ Tissue (sprouted legumes, eggs, SUNLIGHT!)

Vitamin E – Cell Recovery (green vegetables, seeds)

Vitamin K – Vision Health/Blood Clotting (kale)

Vitamins

Useful Antioxidants

+ Polyphenols – Reduce Inflammation (green vegetables, citrus, algae, green tea)

+ Flavonoids – Heart Health (green vegetables, root vegetables)

+ Sulfides – Immune Function (garlic, onion)

+ Curcumin – Cell Recovery (turmeric)

Essential Minerals

Calcium – Bone Health

cruciferous vegetables (broccoli, green leafs), sprouted legumes/seeds/whole grains

Sodium and Chloride (Electrolytes) – Brain Health

green vegetables, sea salt

Potassium (Electrolyte), Molybdenum and Magnesium – Fluid Balance

sprouted legumes/seeds/whole grains, green vegetables

Iron and Copper – Blood Flow

sprouted pulses/seeds/whole grains, green vegetables

Sulfur – Cell Recovery

cruciferous vegetables

Zinc, Phosphorous and Manganese – Cell Recovery

green vegetables, pumpkin seeds

Iodine – Immune Health

sea vegetables, eggs

Selenium – Immune Health

sprouted whole grains, Brazil nuts

Bacteria: A Link In The Polypeptide Chain

Bacteria feed the roots of almost every plant that grows in soil. The same bacteria that live in the soil live in our stomachs, and they feed us too, by breaking food (polypeptides) down into smaller and smaller elements to be effectively used. There are as many of these soil bacteria in our stomachs as there are cells in the entire body.

A healthy body and a healthy planet require a vibrant, thriving bacterial community. Knowing our "roots" helps us know who we are, we are bacteria, bacteria is dirt. Dirt is life!

A Brief History of Life on Earth

To answer the question what was the first food, you must first answer the question, "Who took the first bite?" We can say with fair certainty that every living being has diverged from a common ancestor: the first life form on Earth, let's call her Daisy the Anthropomorphized Amino Acid. Daisy was born 4 billion years ago in a world much different than today. She was in a strange world. For one, her parents were not alive, but not dead, they were organic compounds - abiotic molecules - who met in the heat of the Pre-Cambrian moment. One day, Daisy got hungry. So she learned to use her surroundings to make a scrumptious meal from water, air, minerals and sunlight. It was a tasty morsel that she kept the recipe for, because it was so delicious.

Daisy then learned to wiggle. She wiggled across the primordial mess of Earth until she realized that she was not the only one wiggling around. She was in a community of wigglers. As the community worked together, they learned how to perform functions that build upon one another, until they built a powerhouse. The powerhouse was capable of incredible tasks, like learning to write DNA code. The wiggling community became happy. They sang and danced in their own peculiar way, and after millions of years, the community members all grew a spine, and a heart, and a brain, and flippers, and leaves, and wings, and hands and feet, and emotions. We are living, eating, and breathing the wiggling community. It is our history. The unique intelligence embedded in us is eternal and has always been here. It's up to us to wiggle our way through this life and sing the song of our amino acid ancestors.

Final Notes

You now have the confidence to work in a space of your own, to explore and refine your relationship with yourself through a network of ideas collected in a nebula of community food education. You can share these ideas with anyone, and make them fit to your unique situation by applying the principles here in new ways that you can determine in your home.

This Handbook is a way to understanding the function of fresh food for you, your family, and the collective community of people, plants, animals, fungi, bacteria, air, water drops, and rays of sun that make living on earth as great as it is. Please debate the information in this book at will and make your best judgement for how to interpret this based on experience and wisdom. Enjoy always where you are, and see what you can do to help the world grow around you. Please see a doctor for any underlying conditions and ask them to include a mindfulness practice and whole, real food nutrition into a wellness program for you.

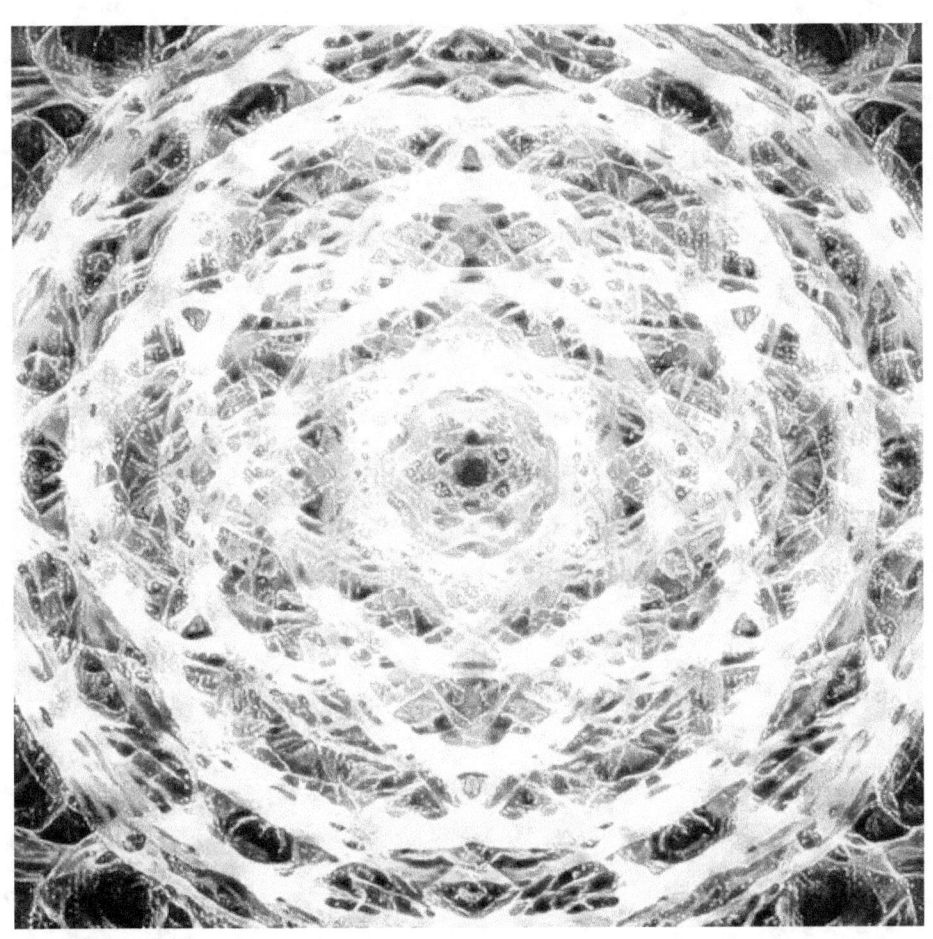

Resource Guide

www.ingramcontent.com/pod-product-compliance
Lightning Source LLC
Chambersburg PA
CBHW062001280526
45787CB00005B/1955